The

Sirt food

Diet

Beginner's Guide for the Celebrities' Diet that Activates the Skinny Gene for Fast Weight Loss and Fat Burn [**7-Day Complete Plan and 30+ Recipes**]

D1601315

By Adele Aidan

Copyright notes

Table of Contents

5

If you open the Kindle preview you can get for **FREE** the **AUDIOBOOK** version of this title with a 30 day Audible trial.

INTRODUCTION TO SIRT FOOD DIET

What is sirtfood?

Sirtfood diet is the new way to quickly lose weight without a radical diet by activating the same "skinny gene" pathways, generally induced by exercise and fasting. Some foods contain chemicals called polyphenols that exert slight stress on our cells, activating genes that mimic the effects of fasting and exercise. Foods rich in polyphenols, such as black cabbage, dark chocolate, and red wine, activate the pathways of sirtuins that influence metabolism, aging, and mood. A diet rich in these body foods initiates weight loss without sacrificing muscles, maintaining optimal health.

Add healthy foods to your diet for effective and sustained weight loss, incredible energy, and radiant health. Turn on your body's fat-burning powers, increase weight loss, and help prevent disease with this easy-to-follow diet developed by nutritional medicine experts. They have demonstrated the impact of milk-based foods. Dark chocolate, coffee, black cabbage: they are all foods that activate sirtuins and activate the so-called "skinny gene" pathways in the body. The Sirtfood diet offers you a simple and healthy way of eating to lose weight, delicious recipes that are easy to prepare, and a maintenance plan for long-term success. The Sirtfood diet is an inclusion diet, not an exclusion diet, and sort foods are available. This is a diet that motivates you to take your knife and fork and enjoy a delicious healthy meal while observing the health benefits and weight loss.

CHAPTER ONE

The science of sirtuins

Sirtuins help regulate cell health. This is what you should know about how they work, what they can do for your body, and why they depend on NAD + to work. Sirtuins are a family of proteins that helps in regulating cellular health. Sirtuins play a major role in regulating cellular homeostasis. Homeostasis involves maintaining the cell in balance. However, sirtuins can only work in the presence of NAD +, nicotinamide adenine dinucleotide, a coenzyme present in all living cells.

How sirtuins regulate cell health with NAD +

Think of your body cells like an office. In the office, many people are working on various tasks with 1 goal: to remain profitable and to carry out the company's mission efficiently for as long as possible. Many pieces in the cells work on various tasks with 1 goal: to stay healthy and work efficiently for as long as possible. Just as the company's priorities change, due to various internal and external factors, the priorities in the cells also change. Someone has to manage the office, regulating what is done when, who will do it and when to change course. In the office, he would be their CEO. In the body, on a cellular level, are your sirtuins.

Sirtuins consist of a family of seven proteins that play a role in cellular health. Sirtuins can only be active in the presence of NAD +, nicotinamide adenine dinucleotide, a coenzyme present in all living cells. NAD + is vital for cellular metabolism and hundreds of other biological processes. If sirtuins are the CEO of a company, then NAD + is the money that pays the CEO and employees' salaries, all while keeping the lights on and paying the rent for the office space. Society and the body cannot function without it. But NAD + levels decrease with age, which also limits the function of sirtuins with age. Unlike everything else, in the human body, it's not that simple. Sirtuins handle everything that happens in your cells.

Sirtuins are proteins. What does it mean?

Sirtuins are a family of proteins. Proteins may look like diet proteins, which are found in beans and meats and, well, in protein shakes, but in this case, we are talking about molecules called proteins, which work in all cells of the body in several different functions. Think of proteins as the departments of a company, each of which focuses on its specific function in coordination with other departments.

A common protein in the body called hemoglobin, which is part of the globin protein family and is responsible for transporting oxygen through the blood. Myoglobin is the counterpart of hemoglobin, and together, they form the globin family. Your body has nearly 60,000 protein families, many departments! And sirtuins are 1 of those families. While hemoglobin is part of a family of two proteins, sirtuins consist of a family of seven.

Three cells out Of the seven sirtuins in the cell, works in the mitochondria, three in the nucleus and 1 in the cytoplasm, and each plays a variety of roles. The basic function of sirtuins, however, is to remove acetyl groups from other proteins. Acetyl groups control specific reactions. They are physical labels on proteins with which other proteins recognize that they will react. If proteins are to be the departments of the cell and DNA the CEO, the acetyl groups are the availability status of each department head. For example, if a protein is available, sirtuin can work with it to make something happen, just as the CEO can work with the head of the department open to make something happen. Sirtuins work with acetyl groups doing what is called deacetylation. This means that they recognize that an acetyl group exists in a molecule and therefore removes the acetyl group, which separates the molecule for their work. 1 way sirtuins work is by removing biological proteins from acetyl groups (deacetylation) such as histones. For example, the deacetylated histones of sirtuins, proteins that are part of a condensed form of DNA called chromatin. Histone is a large, voluminous protein that surrounds DNA. Let us assume it is a Christmas tree, and the DNA chain is the chain of lights. When histones have an acetyl group, the chromatin is open or not rolled up. This chromatin that takes place means that DNA is transcribed, an essential process. But it doesn't need to remain unrolled as it is vulnerable to damage in this position, almost as if the Christmas lights could tangle or the bulbs may be damaged when they are unmanageable or turned on for too long. When histones are deacetylated form sirtuins, the chromatin is closed or tightly closed or injured, which means that gene expression is interrupted or silenced.

We have known sirtuins for 20 years, and their main function was discovered in the 90s. Since then, researchers have come together to study them, identifying their importance and, at the same time, asking questions about what else we can learn about them.

Benefits of Sirtfood

Sirtuins are also involved in several other health benefits like:

To sleep

Activating sirtuins helps your circadian rhythm, making sure you make hormones to sleep and wake up when you should.

Diabetes

Sirtuins make cells more sensitive to insulin, which means they can remove more glucose from the bloodstream. Since insulin resistance is the precursor of both diabetes and weight gain, this can only be good news for your waistline.

Memory

Turmeric has been shown to improve short-term memory and protect against cognitive problems. Prepare your morning juice for a smarter start to the day. But to think of it simply as a weight loss diet is to lose the point. This is a diet that has as much to do with wellness as with life. More energy, clearer skin, greater alertness, and better sleep are the pleasant "side effects" of this way of eating. Sometimes the benefits are even more evident, including cases where the long-term diet has reversed the metabolic disease. Such is their health-enhancing effects that studies show that they are more potent than prescription drugs for preventing chronic diseases, with benefits in diabetes, heart disease, and Alzheimer's, to name a few. It is no wonder that the cultures that consume the most Sirtfood have been the thinnest and healthiest in the world.

Scientific benefits of sirtfood

The latter diet is based on the consumption of foods that could interact with a family of proteins known as sirtuin proteins or SIRT1 - SIRT7. The undoubted appeal of the diet adds to the fact that the best sources presumably include red wine and chocolate, as well as citrus fruits, blueberries, and cabbage.

It looks tasty, and sirtuins are involved in a wide range of cellular processes, including metabolism, aging, and circadian rhythm. This diet is based on part on calorie restriction. nutritionists behind this suggest that the diet "affects the body's ability to burn fat and increases the metabolic system."

What do we know about this special diet? From a scientific point of view, the answer is minimal. Sirtuins help in the regulation of fat and glucose metabolism in response to changes in energy levels. They can also play a role in the effect of calorie restriction on improvements in aging. This may be due to the effects of sirtuins on aerobic (or mitochondrial) metabolism, the decrease in reactive oxygen species (free radicals), and the increase in antioxidant enzymes.

Furthermore, research suggests that transgenic mice with higher SIRT6 levels live significantly longer than wildtype mice and that changes in SIRT6 expression may be relevant in the aging of certain human skin cells. SIRT2 has also been shown to slow down the aging of metazoans (yeasts). It looks impressive, and the diet has some rave reviews, but none of these represent convincing scientific evidence that the Sirtfood diet has similar effects in real people. It would be a colossal overpopulation to assume that laboratory research on mice, yeasts, and human stem cells has an impact on real-world health outcomes, contaminated by a multitude of confounding variables.

CHAPTER TWO

Sirtfood and fat loss

The latest diet cleansing that has thrilled the world follows a scientific approach to combat weight gain.

Here are some problems with body fat.

- Type 2 diabetes

- Hypertension

- Heart disease

- race

- Cancer

- Sleep apnea

- osteoarthritis

- Fatty liver disease

- nephropathy

- Pregnancy problems

Excess fat can increase the risk of many health problems, such as diabetes, heart disease, and certain types of cancer. If you are pregnant, excess weight can cause short and long term health problems for you and your baby.

This fact sheet provides additional information on the links between overweight and many health conditions. It also explains how achieving and maintaining a normal weight can help you, and your loved ones stay healthy with age. The diet is popularized by the use of "Sirt foods," which are some special foods that act by activating some protein chains in the body, known as sirtuins. According to science, these antioxidant agents act as protectors that help delay aging, increase metabolism, and regulate inflammation in the body, thereby helping to lose fat.

Studies have found that this special diet can help people lose up to three pounds in less than a week.

As complex and scientific as this diet looks, the diet encourages you to include some of the most commonly found cooking ingredients, as well as some forgiving foods. Some common foods allowed on this plan include foods such as oranges, dark chocolates, parsley, turmeric, cabbage, and even red wine.

The diet, although considered a fad, focuses on maintaining a restrictive weight loss strategy for a week. While the first three days limit the calorie intake to 1000 kcal (eat three green juices of fresh food and eat). On the remaining days, you are allowed to increase your calorie intake to 1500kcal and consume two meals a day (along with two Sirt food juices). Next, the maintenance phase recommends you eat up to three balanced sirtuin-rich foods, along with an effective weight loss training strategy, which makes it even more sustainable.

Since it is quite restrictive, many remain cautious about the long-term diet plan. The diet limits calorie intake and may lack other necessary nutrients, making it not a long-term sustainable diet plan for weight loss.

Sirtuins and exercises

Exercise is any movement that makes the muscles work and requires the body to burn calories.

There are lots of physical activities, such as swimming, running, running, walking, and dancing, just to name a few. Being active has proven to have many health benefits, both physical and mental. It can also help you live longer.

Here are the ten best ways in which regular exercise benefits your body and brain.

1. It can make you feel happier

Exercise has been shown to improve mood and decrease the feeling of depression, anxiety, and stress.

It manifests changes in the parts of the brain that helps in regulating stress and anxiety. It also increases the brain sensitivity to the hormones serotonin and norepinephrine, which relieve feelings of depression.

Exercise can also increase the production of endorphins, which are known to help produce positive sensations and reduce pain perception.

Also, exercise has been shown to reduce symptoms in people with anxiety. It also helps them become more aware of their mental state and practice distracting their fears.

Oddly enough, it doesn't matter how intense your training is. Your mood can also benefit from exercise regardless of the intensity of physical activity.

2. It can help with weight loss.

Studies have shown that inactivity is a key factor in weight gain and obesity. To fully grasp the effect of exercise on weight reduction, it is important to understand the relationship between exercise and energy expenditure.

3. It is good for muscles and bones.

Exercise plays a major role in building and maintaining strong muscles and bones.

Physical activity, such as lifting weights, can stimulate muscle development if combined with sufficient protein intake.

This is so because exercise helps in releasing hormones that promote muscle capacity to absorb amino acids. This helps them to grow and reduces their breakdown.

As we age, they tend to lose muscle mass and function, which can lead to injury and disability. Regular physical activity is significant to reduce muscle loss and maintain strength with age.

Plus, exercise helps increase bone density when you're younger, as well as preventing osteoporosis later in life. Interestingly, high-impact exercises, like gymnastics or running, or odd-impact sports, like soccer and basketball, have been shown to promote higher bone density than non-impact sports such as swimming and cycling.

4. It can increase energy levels.

Exercise can be a real energy boost for healthy people, as well as for those with various medical conditions. A study found that six weeks of regular exercise reduced feelings of fatigue for 36 healthy people who reported persistent fatigue.

Additionally, exercise can significantly increase energy levels for people with chronic fatigue syndrome and other serious illnesses.

Exercise appears to be more effective in fighting CFS than other treatments, including passive therapies like relaxation and stretching, or no treatment at all.

Also, exercise has shown to increase energy levels in people with progressive diseases such as cancer, HIV / AIDS, and multiple sclerosis.

5. It can reduce the risk of having chronic diseases.

Lack of regular physical activity is a leading cause of chronic illness.

Regular exercise improves insulin sensitivity, cardiovascular fitness, and body composition, but at the same time reduce blood pressure and fat levels in the blood.

Conversely, lack of regular exercise, even in the short term, can lead to significant increases in abdominal fat, increasing the risk of having type 2 diabetes, heart disease, and premature death.

Therefore, regular physical activity is recommended to reduce abdominal fat and the risk of developing these diseases.

6. It can help in skin health.

Your skin can be affected by the oxidative stress on your body. This can damage the internal structures of the skin. Although intense and full physical activity contributes to oxidative damage, regular moderate exercise can increase the body's production of natural antioxidants, helping to protect cells.

Similarly, exercise can stimulate blood flow and induce adaptations of skin cells that can help delay the onset of skin aging.

7. It can help the brain and memory.

Exercise can also improve brain function and protect memory and thinking skills. For starters, it increases the heart rate, promoting the flow of blood and oxygen to the brain. It can also stimulate the production of body hormones, which can improve the growth of brain cells.

Also, the ability of exercise to prevent chronic diseases can translate into benefits for the brain, since its function can be affected by these diseases. Frequent physical activity is particularly important in the elderly since aging, combined with oxidative stress and inflammation, promotes changes in the structure and function of the brain. Exercise has been shown to grow the hippocampus, a vital part of the brain for memory and learning—and this increases the mental ability in the elderly.

However, exercise has been shown to reduce changes in the brain that can cause Alzheimer's disease and schizophrenia.

8. It can help with good relaxation and sleep quality.

Exercising regularly can help you relax and sleep better.

Regarding the quality of sleep, the energy depletion that occurs during exercise stimulates the recovery processes during sleep.

Additionally, the increase in body temperature that occurs during exercise is believed to improve sleep quality by helping you decrease during sleep.

Lots of studies on the effects of exercise on sleep have gotten similar conclusions. 1 study found that 150 minutes of moderate to vigorous activity per week can provide up to 65% improvement in sleep quality (40).

Another showed that 16 weeks of regular exercise improved sleep quality and helped 17 people with insomnia sleep more and more soundly than the control group. It also helped them to feel more energetic during the day.

Also, regular exercise seems to be beneficial for the elderly, who tend to suffer from sleep disorders.

You can be flexible with the type of exercise you choose. It seems that aerobic exercise alone or aerobic exercise combined with resistance training can also help sleep quality.

9. Can reduce pain

Chronic pain can be debilitating. However, exercise can help reduce it. In fact, for several years, the recommendation for the treatment of chronic pain was rest and inactivity. However, recent studies have shown that exercise also helps to relieve chronic pain. A review of several studies shows that exercise helps participants with chronic pain reduce pain and improve quality of life.

Studies have shown that exercise helps to manage pain associated with various health conditions, including chronic low back pain, fibromyalgia, and chronic soft tissue shoulder disorder, to name a few.

Additionally, physical activity can also increase pain tolerance and decrease pain perception.

10. It can promote a better sex life.

Exercise has been shown to help in increasing sexual desire. Regular exercise can also strengthen the cardiovascular system, improve blood circulation, tl muscles, and improve flexibility, all of which can improve your sex life.

Physical activity also helps to improve sexual performance and sexual pleasure, as well as increase the frequency of sexual activity.

Sirtfood and muscles: muscular activities that you can add to your sirtuin's diet.

1. Stretch up

Stand up straight with your legs straight, making sure your knees aren't locked. Slowly lower your torso to the floor, then walk your hands forward. Once in the flexed position, begin to take small steps so that your feet meet your hands. Keep bothering you for 4-6 reps.

2. Tuck jump

Stand up with your knees slightly bent, then jump as high as possible, pretend Jeremy Lin is watching! Bring your knees up to your chest as you extend your arms out. Land with your knees slightly bent and jumped again quickly (on top of it)!

3. Tracking

Embrace that inner brown bear. Starting with your hands and knees, lift your toes, squeeze the core, and slowly stretch forward with your right arm and right knee, followed by the left side. Continue the scan for 8-10 reps (or until you turn off your roommates).

4. Alpinist

Start on your hands and knees. Place your left foot forward, directly under your chest, while stretching your right leg. Keeping his hands on the ground and his core tight, he jumps and changes legs.

The left leg should now extend behind you, with the right knee forward. The next? Everest.

5. Plyometric push-ups

Ready to get some air? Start on a well-padded surface and perform a traditional flex. In an explosive motion, push up enough to lift yourself off the ground (and hang ten for a second!). Once you have returned to the mainland, go immediately to the next representative.

6. Climb the ladder with your biceps curl

Turn those scales into a cardio machine; you don't need a magic wand. Grab some weights (or household items) and quickly go up and down the stairs while simultaneously doing bicep curls to work your entire body.

7. Prone disorder

Start on all fours with your core busy. Move your hands slowly forward, staying alert but not moving forward. Then gradually return your hands to the starting position, maintaining stability and balance. This dance comes later.

8. Burpee

1 of the most effective exercises for the whole body, start in a low position, and squat with your hands on the floor. Then return your feet to a flexed position.

Complete a push-up, then immediately return your feet to a squatting position. Jump as high as possible before bending down and returning to the push-up portion of the show.

9. Plank

No, luckily, we are not walking on the table. Lie down flat and place your forearms on the ground and hands clasped. Stretch your legs behind you and lift your toes. Keep your back straight, squeeze the core, and hold for 30 to 60 seconds (or until you can hang it up).

10. Plank to push up

Start in a plank position. Gently place 1 hand at a time on the ground to lift it into a flexed position, with your back straight and the core hooked. Return 1 arm at a time to the bridge position (forearms on the ground). Repeat for several turns, alternating the arm that makes the first movement.

11. Sit on the wall

Who needs a chair when there is a wall?

Slowly slide your back along the wall until your thighs are parallel to the floor. Ensure your knees are directly above your ankles and keep your back straight. Continue for 60 seconds per set (or how long it takes to turn those legs into jelly). Do you need more fire? Add some bicep curls.

12. Lunge

Stand up with your hands, placed on your hips and feet at the width of your hips. Bring your right leg forward and slowly lower your body until your left (rear) knee is close to or touches the ground and bend at least 90 degrees. Go back to the starting position and repeat on the other side. For a change, try backing off the lunge.

13. Clock in thrust

Time for a challenge. Complete a traditional lunge forward, then take a big step to the right and descend again. Finish the semicircle with a lunge back, then return to your feet. And all this is 1 repetition! Aim for ten reps, then switch legs.

14. Sink to row

Start by making a normal lunge. Instead of returning that leg forward to the starting position, lift it off the ground by raising your arms. The leg should remain bent about 90 degrees. Add weights to provide warmth.

15. Gun squats

A gun permit may not be required for this, but it's not a joke yet.

Stand with your arms straight in front of your body. Raise your right leg, flex your right ankle, and push your hips back. Lower your body while keeping your right leg elevated. Hold (have fun with that), then stand up again.

16. Leap jump

Ready to amaze some friends? Stand with your feet together and launch forward with your right foot. Jump high, pushing your arms forward, keeping your elbows bent.

While in the air, change your legs and land in a lunge with the opposite leg forward. Repeat and keep changing legs. Try making 10!

17.Reverence lunge

We will show some respect. When throwing, pull the left leg behind the right leg, bending the knees and lowering the hips until the right thigh is almost parallel to the floor. Remember to keep your torso upright and your hips squared.

18.squat

Stand with your feet parallel or rotated 15 degrees, whichever is more comfortable. Start to bend slowly by bending your hips and knees until your thighs are at least parallel to the floor.

Make sure your heels don't rise off the floor. Press your heels to get back on your feet.

19.one-leg deadlift

Start standing with your feet together. Raise your right leg slightly. Lower your arms and torso as you lift your right leg behind you. Place your left knee slightly bent and reach your arms as close to the ground as possible.

20. Squats reach and jump

Ready to add some dynamism (and cardio) to that squat? Perform a normal squat, but jump immediately, stretching your arms. Aim for 15 reps, then take a breather before the next set.

21. Chair in a squatting pose

Stand upright while your feet shoulder-width are apart and perform a squat until your thighs are parallel to the floor while raising your arms. Straighten your legs, then lift your right knee while swinging your left arm from your right knee. Get up again and repeat on the other side.

22. Leg lift quadrupled

Start with your hands and knees, with your back flat and the core hooked. Lift your left leg back, stopping when your foot is at hip height, and your thigh is parallel to the floor.

Swing as long as possible, then lift your bottom right tip off the floor, squeezing your butt, back and abs, try to be elegant here! Hold for up about 10 seconds, then switch legs.

23. Step-up

Find a step or bench. Place your right foot on the raised surface. Move forward until the right leg is straight (do it for Channing!), Then return to the starting position. Repeat, while aiming for 10-12 reps on each side.

24. Breeding of calves

From an upright position, slowly rise on your toes, keeping your knees straight and heels raised off the ground. Wait a moment, then go back. Aaa and repeat. Try to stand on something high (like a step) to get a wider range of motion.

25. Standard flex

There is a reason why this is a classic. With your hands apart at shoulder width, keep your feet flexed at the distance of your hips and squeeze the core. Bend your elbows until your chest touches the floor, then push up. Make sure to keep your elbows close to your body. That's one!

26. Dolphin push-ups

Start with Dolphin Pose (think of the downward-facing dog pose with your elbows on the ground). Bend forward, lowering your shoulders until your head is on your hands. Push up with your arms and go back to the starting position. The ocean is not necessary.

27. Increase in the contralateral limb

Seems classy, huh? Here is the break: lie on your stomach with your arms open and your palms facing each other. Slowly lift an arm a few inches off the floor, keeping it straight without turning your shoulders and keeping your head and torso steady. Hold the position, then lower the arm. Repeat on the other side.

For an additional challenge, raise the opposite leg a few inches above the floor simultaneously.

28.Donkey kick

It is time to embrace that wild side. Start in a flexed position with your legs together. Squeeze the core and kick the two legs in the air with the knees bent, reaching the feet towards the buttocks. Try to land gently when you return to your starting position.

29.Manual push

Fair warning: this move is for professionals. Stand upright against the wall. Bend your elbows, making an inverted flex so that your head moves to the floor and your legs stay against the wall. Noob? Find a friend to see you, safety first!

30.Judo push-ups

From a flexed position, lift those hips up and with a quick movement: hai-yah! - try to use your arms to lower the front of your body until your chin is close to the floor. Slide your head and shoulders upward and lower your hips, keeping your knees off the ground. Reverse the movement to return to the raised position of the hip. Try repeating for 30 to 60 seconds.

31.Reverse

For DIY weights, take two cans or bottles of water. Stand upright, and place 1 foot in front of the other, and the front knee slightly bent.

With the palms facing each other and the abdominals contracted, tilted slightly forward from the waist and extended the arms to the sides, squeezing the shoulder blades. To repeat.

32. Superman

Do you want superpowers? Lie flat on your stomach with your arms and legs stretched out. Keeping your torso as firm as possible, simultaneously raise your arms and legs to form a small curve in your body. Optional layer.

33. Dip triceps

Sit on the floor next to a step or bench, with your knees slightly bent. Grab the edge of the raised surface and stretch your arms.

Bend your arms at a 90-degree angle and straighten again as your heels push towards the floor. For a little more fire, extend your right arm as you raise your left leg.

34. Push-up diamond

Rhianna would approve it! Stand in a flexed position with your diamond-shaped hands so that your thumbs and index fingers touch each other. So do push-ups!

This hand position will give those triceps extras (burning) love.

35. Boxer

It is time to make Muhammad Ali proud. Stand with your feet shoulder-width apart and bend your knees forward until your torso is almost parallel to the floor. Keep your elbows inside and extend 1 arm forward and the other back. Hug your arms back and swap your arms like you're in the ring!

36. Shoulder stabilization series (I-Y-T-W-O)

Well, it may sound ridiculous, but stay with us. Lie flat on your stomach and stretch your arms over your head and palms facing each other. Move your arms in every letter formation. Give me a Y; you know what you want!

37. Arm rims

Remember the physical education course? Stand with your arms extended to the sides, perpendicular to your torso. Turn slowly clockwise about 1 foot in diameter for 20-30 seconds. Then reverse the movement, going counterclockwise.

38. Headquarters L

Remove the load (well, not exactly). Sit with your legs extended, and your feet flexed. Place your hands on the ground and slightly around your torso. Raise your hips off the ground and hold for 5 seconds and release. To repeat!

39. Rotational push-up

Standard push-ups don't cut it? First, after returning to an initial lifting position, turn your body to the right and extend your right hand upward, forming a T with your arms and torso. Go back to the starting position, do a normal push-up, then turn left.

40.Frenetic kick

Lie on your back with your arms to the sides and palms down. With your legs extended, lift your heels about 6 inches off the floor. Make quick and small pulses up and down with your legs, keeping the core busy. Keep kicking him for a consecutive minute!

41.Prone Dynamic Board

Starting from a normal table position, raise your hips as high as possible, then lower them. Repeat this movement for as long as possible. Make sure your back stays straight, and your hips don't fall.

42.Side

Lie on your back and roll on 1 side. Go up to 1 foot and elbow. Make sure the hips are raised, and the core is hooked. Hold on for 30 to 60 seconds, or as long as possible!

43.Russian twist

Sit on the floor with your knees bent and your feet together, raised a few inches off the floor. With your back tilted 45 degrees to the floor, swing your arms from side to side with a twisting motion.

In this scenario, the slow and steady wins the race: the slower the curve, the deeper the burn. Do you already feel like a fitness czar?

44.Bicycle

Lie with your back while your knees bent and your hands behind your head. Bring your knees to your chest. Place your right elbow towards your left knee when your right leg is straightened. Continue alternating the sides as if you were pedaling a bicycle. Keep your helmet in the closet.

45.Crunch

Before crowning Cap'n Crunch, remember: the shape is the key. Lie with your back while your knees bent and your feet flat on the floor, with your hands behind your head, slightly lower your chin.

Remove your head and shoulders from the floor while working on your core. Continue to twist until the upper back comes off the mat. Press and hold briefly, then slowly lower your upper body to the ground.

46.Segmental rotation

Let's aim for those obliques! Lie with your back while your knees bent and your heart tight, let your knees gradually drop to the left until you feel good to stretch. Hold for 5 seconds, go back to the center, and repeat on the right.

47.Bridge over the shoulders

Lie with your back while your knees are bent and your feet apart at the width of your hips. Place your arms on the sides and raise your spine and hips.

Lift 1 leg, keeping the core tight. Slowly lower your leg, then lift again. Try doing ten reps per leg, then lower your spine to the ground.

48. Abdominal 1 leg press

Lie with your back flat, with your knees bent and your feet flat on the floor. Squeeze your abs and lift your right leg, with your knee bent at a 90-degree angle.

Push your right hand over the raised knee, using the soul to create pressure between the hand and the knee. Hold for 5 seconds, then lower your back. Repeat with your left hand and knee.

49. Double-leg abdominal press

Two legs are twice as fun! Follow the same summary for the 1 leg press (see # 48), but lift both legs at the same time, pushing your hands against your knees.

50. Sprinter situp

Do you want to be a speed demon without getting up from the ground? Lie on your back with your legs stretched out and your arms on the sides, your elbows bent at a 90-degree angle. Now sit down and bring your left knee towards your right elbow. Go back to the starting position. Repeat on the other side.

Your body gives out energy in three different ways: digesting food, exercising, and maintaining bodily functions such as heart rate and breathing.

During the diet, reduced calorie intake will lower the metabolic rate, slowing down weight loss. On the contrary, frequent exercise has been shown to increase metabolic rate, which burns more calories and helps you lose weight.

Also, studies have shown that combining aerobic exercise with resistance training can maximize fat loss and maintain muscle mass, which is essential for maintaining weight.

For some people, it may not be so difficult to lose weight or maintain a healthy weight. However, the Sirtfood diet can help those who are struggling. But how about combining the Sirtfood diet with exercise? Is it advisable to completely avoid exercise or introduce it once the diet has started?

It is important to find healthy eating and feasible exercise regimens that don't deprive you of anything you like and don't require you to exercise all week. The Sirtfood diet does exactly that. The idea is that some foods will activate the "skinny gene" pathways, which are generally activated through fasting and exercise. The great news is that some foods and drinks, including dark chocolate and red wine, contain chemicals called polyphenols that activate genes that mimic the effects of exercise and fasting.

CHAPTER THREE

Exercise for the first few weeks.

In the first week or two of the diet in which the calorie intake is reduced, it would be wise to stop or reduce exercise as the body adapts to fewer calories. Give attention to your body, and if you feel tired or have less energy than usual, do not exercise. Instead, be sure to stay focused on the principles that apply to a healthy lifestyle, such as including adequate daily levels of fiber, protein, and fruit and vegetables.

Once the diet becomes a lifestyle

When you exercise, it is essential to consume protein, ideally 1 hour after training. Protein repairs muscles after exercise reduce pain and can aid recovery. There are lots of recipes that include a protein that will be perfect for consumption after exercises, such as chili with meat or chicken and coleslaw with turmeric. If you want to prefer something lighter, you can try cranberry smoothie and add some protein powder for an added benefit. The type of exercise you will do will depend on you, but home workouts will allow you to choose the best time to exercise, the types of exercises that are suitable for you, and that are short and convenient.

The Sirtfood diet is a great way to change your eating habits, lose weight, and feel healthier. The first few weeks can put you to the test, but it's essential to check which foods are best to eat and right for you. Be good to yourself in the first few weeks as your body adjusts and exercise calmly if you choose to do it. If you are the type that carries out intense exercise, it is possible you can continue reasonably or check your physical condition based on the change in diet. As with any change in diet and exercise, it is about the person and how hard they can feel.

Sirtuins and Diseases

Sirtuins influence various cellular processes. Mounting evidence has recently highlighted their involvement in many diseases.

Adults are more likely to develop certain diet-related illnesses, such as hypertension (high blood pressure), heart disease, cancer, and osteoporosis. Older adults are more likely to request a change in diet to control the disease than younger adults, but the diet must still reflect the preferences of the older adult. For the elderly, the diet should be tailored to the person rather than changing the person's eating behavior. Food should not be denied simply because a person is older.

Hypertension

An estimated 40-50% of adults in the United States are "at-risk" of developing hypertension. Untreated hypertension can lead to:

- race.

- Renal insufficiency.

- Myocardial infarction.

- Heart failure.

In general, a high sodium intake (but not proven) is believed to increase the risk of high blood pressure. In some people, other risk factors include:

- heritage.

- Obesity.

- Fatigue.

Weight loss can help lower high blood pressure. Some people can reduce high blood pressure by limiting sodium intake. Others can significantly lower their blood pressure by increasing calcium intake. Those who are sensitive to salt appear to be particularly sensitive to increased calcium intake.

Some interactions between medications and nutrients can result in additional vitamin or mineral needs for older adults. However, some people need to control hypertension using the medication, which is generally a diuretic that also wastes potassium (decreases retention). Potassium is important for:

- water balance.

- Muscle contraction.

- Maintenance of a normal heartbeat.

Although a doctor may prescribe a potassium supplement, it is an expensive and unpleasant taste. The surest way to protect potassium from the body, without providing more sodium than a hypertensive patient's diet would allow, is to include a large number of fruits and fruit juices in your diet. Fruits are the only foods rich in potassium and generally prepared and consumed without adding sodium.

Heart disease

Heart attacks are responsible for death and disease all over the world. The root cause of heart attacks is a disease called "arteriosclerosis," which is the accumulation of "plaque" or "crude" (cholesterol, fatty deposits, and other substances) in the inner lining of the artery walls. This build-up constricts the arteries until they become blocked so that blood cannot flow. This can cause death or damage to part of the heart muscle, a heart attack.

Many factors are associated with heart disease. For example, a smoker is statistically more likely to develop cardiovascular disease and die of a heart attack or stroke than a non-smoker; therefore, smoking is a "risk factor" for heart disease. Other factors associated with increased risk are:

- gender (being a man).

- Inheritance (includes diabetes).

- Hypertension.

- Lack of exercise.

- Obesity.

- Fatigue.

- high blood cholesterol

Risk factors are powerful predictors of heart disease. Three risk factors with greater intensity have been studied: smoking, hypertension, and high cholesterol.

Millions of dollars have been spent, and decades of research have been conducted to determine exactly what causes heart disease. Although hundreds of researchers have shown positive results from research on risk factors, it is not yet possible to determine the exact causes of heart disease. In summary, although diet and nutrition are the focus of attention in heart disease, it is important to have a Better view of the problem. Nutrition is not the only factor involved.

Furthermore, there is recent evidence that arteriosclerosis begins in childhood. Some studies have shown that plaque buildup can progress slowly in coronary artery disease in adulthood.

Cholesterol

Cholesterol is produced in the liver and is sent through the bloodstream to all parts of the body. Cholesterol is necessary for the body to:

- producing hormones (such as vitamin D and sex hormones).

- Mold covers that protect nerve fibers.

- Create strong cell membranes.

The liver also uses cholesterol to produce the bile acids necessary to digest fats. In 1 day, the liver produces 1,000 milligrams of cholesterol to meet the body's needs.

The typical diet offers around 600 milligrams of cholesterol per day, in addition to what the liver produces. Although this is much less than what the liver produces on its own, it can exceed the body's ability to contain the amount of cholesterol circulating in the blood. Therefore, blood cholesterol levels increase.

Cholesterol is carried through the bloodstream in packages called lipoproteins. High-density lipoproteins, or HDLs, are of the "good" type; They remove cholesterol from the body's cells and tissues in the liver to sweat it. Low-density lipoproteins, or LDL, are the "bad" type responsible for depositing cholesterol on the walls of the arteries.

The amount of cholesterol circulating in the body's blood is affected by more than the amount of cholesterol consumed. It is also influenced by the amount and type of fat consumed. In particular, diets rich in saturated fat tend to increase the level of cholesterol in the blood, while polyunsaturated and monounsaturated fats help reduce it.

The more cholesterol in a person's blood, the greater the chance that something will build upon the inner walls of the body's arteries like "plaques." These plates get bigger and bigger. The width of the blood vessels narrows until the clot completely stops any blood flow through the artery. If the artery leads to the heart, a heart attack can occur because the heart muscle has not received the essential oxygen supply necessary to do its job. If the artery leads to the brain, a stroke can occur. The arteries in the legs can also become blocked; Painful muscle spasms can occur from the slightest exercise because the muscles don't get enough oxygen.

Studies have confirmed that the amount and type of fat and the amount of cholesterol consumed directly affect a person's risk of dying from coronary heart disease prematurely. There is some evidence that a reversal of arteriosclerosis can occur in people who reduce the amount of saturated fat and cholesterol.

Regular exercise can promote a healthier heart in two ways:

- keeps body weight in a desirable range.

- It can increase the level of "good" cholesterol (HDL) in the body.

Remember that fats and cholesterol are not the only dietary components that can influence a person's risk of developing heart disease. Other factors implicated by research studies include:

- The hardness of the water.

- Amount of sugar in the diet.

- Amount of dietary fiber in the diet.

- Various vitamins.

- Caffeine.

- Others.

It is not possible to indicate a particular individual and predict what effect the diet will have on that person's chances of developing heart disease. The genetic predisposition of an individual influence the extent of the damage that the environment can cause.

Cancer

The same high-fat diet associated with heart disease can also increase the risk of developing some types of cancer, the leading life-threatening tumor in the United States.

Breast cancer, the leading killer of women's cancer.

Obesity is a risk factor associated with a high risk of developing breast and endometrial cancers. Chemical reactions in body fat cause the formation of substances that act similarly to female sex hormones; They can stimulate the growth of breast and endometrial cancers.

Among the Japanese, who eat little fat of any kind, breast and colon cancers are rare. Studies have shown that when a diet contains high amounts of fat and cholesterol, intestinal bacteria break these foods down into substances that can directly cause cancer or promote the action of other carcinogenic chemicals. Since such diets generally contain fat and fibrous foods, the stool tends to concentrate and stay longer in the colon than usual; there is more exposure to carcinogens.

Also, some of the substances produced by cholesterol from intestinal bacteria can mimic the action of female sex hormones. This can promote cancer growth in hormone-sensitive tissues, such as the breast and endometrium (lining of the uterus).

Osteoporosis

. It is the leading cause of "narrowing" in height and bone fractures among the elderly. Starting in the 1920s for women and a little later for men, calcium is gradually lost from the bones. It results in a shortening and weakening of the long bones and greatly increases a woman's susceptibility to fractures. This loss of calcium is accelerated in women after menopause. Over 50 years of age, 25-30% of women and 15-20% of men suffer from a shortening of the spine due to osteoporosis.

Osteoporosis affects 1 in four women after menopause. It causes a loss of height with age due to the collapse of the spinal vertebrae, producing the characteristic "widow's hump." Osteoporosis is the leading cause of debilitating hip and wrist fractures that commonly affect older women. It can also be a factor of bone loss in the jaws; it eventually leads to tooth loss due to periodontal disease.

Menopausal women ages three to six can help prevent bone loss by increasing calcium intake and exercising a lot. Although older women use large amounts of calcium supplements, evidence shows that such supplements can prevent or stop the progress of osteoporosis in some, but not all, people. Calcium in the diet (calcium from food) is much better absorbed and used by the body than supplements. However, no supplement can replace the calcium lost from the bones; at best, it can slow down deterioration even further. Therefore, prevention is critical.

Fluorine is also important for bone strength. Osteoporosis is significantly less common in communities that receive fluoridated water; This suggests that fluoride protects against the disease and the accompanying fractures. Fluoride works with calcium in the bone and helps prevent common calcium loss after middle age.

Other factors, in addition to the amount of calcium consumed, influence the amount of this mineral absorbed by the body. Below is a partial list.

Active vitamin D is necessary for calcium to be absorbed through the intestinal tract; the elderly make less of this active form of vitamin D.

Vitamin C improves the absorption of calcium, as well as lactose (milk sugar).

Overeating protein or fat interferes with calcium absorption; it greatly increases the amount of calcium lost by the body.

Inactivity accelerates the loss of calcium; Exercise for life helps prevent bone loss with age.

Some foods contain substances that bind to the calcium in these foods to prevent mineral absorption. These substances include:

oxalic acid in spinach, Swiss chard, Swiss chard, and rhubarb; is

Phytic acid in whole bran. However, it is believed that this link does not seriously interfere with the amount of calcium the body receives.

Too much phosphorus can increase the need for calcium and thus create a deficiency even if there is an adequate amount of calcium in the diet. This can be a problem among adults who consume few or no dairy products or among adolescents who drink too much carbonated (phosphorous-rich) drink.

The loss of estrogen at menopause greatly accelerates the loss of calcium from a woman's bones.

Although SirT1 has been extensively studied, a better understanding of its involvement in pathogenesis is needed. Many questions remain unaddressed, such as the role of other sirtuins and their role. More research is needed to provide clearer perspectives. The development of powerful sirtuin modulators can reverse the disease process and possibly extend the duration of healthy human life.

Sirtuins and genome stability

Some sirtuins (SirT1, 2, 3, 6) are related to the regulation of chromatin since they are responsible for regulating two modifications of post-translational histones crucial for the structure of chromatin. SirT1 is accountable for the formation of heterochromatin through a deacetylation process. Histone deacetylation can alter histone methylation, thus improving overall transcriptional repression.

CHAPTER FOUR

How to Create A Sirtfood Diet That Works

Are you enjoing this book? If so, I'd be really happy if you could leave a short review on Amazon, it means a lot to me! Thank you

The Sirtfood diet consists of two phases of a total of three weeks. You can then continue to "saturate" your diet by including as many meat products as possible in your meals. Specific recipes for these two stages can be found in this book. Meals are packed with sirt foods but contain other ingredients besides the "Top 20 sirt foods". Most of the elements and prepared dishes are easy to find. However, three of the distinctive ingredients needed for these two stages - matcha green tea powder, wild celery, and buckwheat - can be expensive or hard to find.

A large part of the diet is the green juice, which should be prepared one to three times a day.

You will wish a juicer (a blender will not work) and a kitchen range as the ingredients are listed by weight. The recipe is below:

Sirtfood Green Juice

Ingredients

75 grams / 2,5 ounce of cabbage

30 grams / 1 ounce rocket

5 grams / 1 teaspoon of parsley

Two celery stalks

1 cm (0.5 inches) of ginger

half green apple

partly a lemon

half a teaspoon of matcha green tea

Instructions

Squeeze all the ingredients except the green tea powder and lemon and pour them into a glass. Squeeze the lemon by hand and then mix the lemon juice and green tea powder into its sauce.

Stage one

The first phase lasts seven days and includes a reduction in calories and plenty of green juice. The goal is to restart weight loss and is said to help you lose 3.2 kg in 7 days.

During the first three days of the first phase, caloric intake is limited to 1,000 calories. Drink three green juices a day plus a meal. You can choose from the recipes in the book every day, which include all fish dishes as the central part of the meal.Examples of meals include poorly glazed tofu, sirt food omelet, or fried shrimp with buckwheat noodles.On days 4-7 of the first phase, caloric intake increased to 1,500. This includes two green juices a day and two more sirt food-rich foods, which you can choose from the book.

Stage two

Phase two lasts two weeks. During this "maintenance" phase, you have to keep losing weight consistently.There is no definite calorie limit for this phase. Instead, eat three meals full of sirt food and 1 green juice a day. Again, meals are chosen from the recipes in the book.

After the diet

You can repeat these two procedures as many times as you want to lose more weight.However, we recommend that you continue to "satiate" your diet after completing these steps by regularly including blueberry foods in your meals.

There are several Sirtfood diet books rich in sirtfood-rich recipes. You can also include sirt foods in your diet as a snack or in the methods you already use.

How to Make the Sirtfood Plan

You may have heard of the Sirtfood plan before, especially since singer Adele reportedly lost 50 pounds after the program, but do you know what it is? The nutrition plan defines the 20 foods that activate the so-called "lean genes" increasing your metabolism and energy levels. He even claims that he could lose 7 kg in 7 days.The diet plan changes the way you eat healthily. It may sound like a name that is not easy to use, but you will hear a lot about it.Since the "Sirt" in Sirtfoods is a shortcut for sirtuin genes, a group of genes nicknamed "skinny genes" that, frankly, work like magic.

Eating these foods, plan makers, nutritionists Aidan Goggins and Glen Matten, activate these genes and "mimic the effects of calorie constraint, fasting, and exercise." It enables a recycling process in the body, "which removes cellular debris and the condition that builds up over time and causes health problems and loss of vitality," the authors write.

What happens after you finish the Sirt food diet

The Sirtfood diet is not designed to be a single "diet," but rather a way of life. We recommend continuing to follow a Sirtfood-rich diet after completing the first three weeks and continuing to drink green juice daily. Since the release of their original book, the authors of The Sirtfood Diet have continued to publish The Sirtfood Diet Recipe Book, with recipes for many other Sirtfood-rich meals, recipes for alternatives to green juice, and other tips and tricks for Sirt Food Diet. There are also some Sirtfood dessert recipes! The authors of The Sirtfood Diet suggest that steps 1 and 2 can be repeated if necessary to improve health and when they are out of control.

Sirtuin and Cancer

Findings in sirtuins have grown in the last decade, mainly due to their critical roles in different biological processes, like regulation of gene expression, control of metabolic processes, apoptosis and cell survival, DNA repair, development, neuroprotection and inflammation. Sirtuins control many important functions and are involved in various pathologies, such as metabolic diseases, neurodegenerative disorders, and cancer.

SirT1 is significantly upregulated in various cancers, including acute myeloid leukemia (AML), prostate, colon, and skin cancer..

Sirtuin and aging diseases.

Sirtuins are believed to be handy in metabolic diseases, neurodegeneration, and aging.

It is known that overexpression of Sir2 (or its orthologs) can prolong the life of the organism in a wide range of lower eukaryotes). The Sirt2 function is often related to calorie restriction. The link between the role of sirtuins, calorie restriction, and longevity has been first described in S. cerevisiae. In yeast, calorie restriction leads to an increase in replicative life. No extension of shelf life was observed in Sir2-free yeasts. Currently, the role of sirtuins in regulating the life expectancy of mammals is still unclear. However, considering that sirtuins are an evolutionary family of conserved proteins, it is correct to speculate about their role in modulating aging-related processes in higher organisms. In humans, the aging process is accompanied by erosion of the telomeres. SirT1 and SirT6 have an important role in both telomere maintenance and function and the aging process. Recent studies have shown that reduction or elimination of SirT6 causes telomeric dysfunction and end-to-end chromosome fusions. The symptoms displayed in the absence of SirT6 are similar to those caused by an early aging disease known as Werner syndrome. To date, not much is known about other sirtuins, but no evidence suggests their involvement in telomere function, formation, and stability.

Many studies have shown that the pathogenesis of neurodegenerative diseases includes large changes and the participation of multiple biochemical pathways. Sirtuins play a critical role in numerous neurodegenerative disease models. Numerous reports support SirT1's role in axonal protection from damage in animal models of Vallerand degenerative disease.

Sirtuin modulators

Sirtuins play a key role in various pathologies. Of recent, a great deal of research interest has focused on the identification of small chemical compounds that modulate these proteins. To date, many sirtuin inhibitors have been proposed for therapy against neurodegenerative diseases and cancer. Numerous inhibitors have been discovered and characterized in recent years. In addition to nicotinamide, the physiological inhibitor of sirtuin, some specific inhibitors have been proposed.

Can you eat meat with the Sirtfood diet?

The answer is a resounding yes. The diet plan not only includes the consumption of a healthy portion of meat but recommends that proteins be an essential inclusion in a Sirtfood-based diet to achieve maximum benefit in maintaining metabolism and reducing exhaustion. Muscle common in most diet programs. Heavy meat diet (we still remember the halitosis of the Atkins diet); in reality, it is very vegetarian. It is aimed at almost everyone, which makes it such a sensible choice.

Leucine is an amino acid present in proteins, which effectively integrates and improves the actions of Sirtfoods. This means the best way to eat Sirtfoods is to combine them with a chicken breast, a fillet, or another source of leucine such as fish.

Poultry meats can be eaten freely (because it is an excellent source of protein, B vitamins, potassium, and phosphorus). Red meat is another excellent source of protein, iron, and can eat up to three times (750 g / 26.5 oz gross weight) per week.

Phase 1 and phase 2 of sirtfood.

Phase 1

The first phase lasts seven days and involves a reduction in calories and a lot of green juice. Its goal is to restart weight loss and is claimed to help you lose 3.2 kg in 7 days.

During the first three days of the first phase, calorie intake is limited to 1,000 calories. Drink three green juices a day plus a meal. Every day you can choose from the recipes in the book, which include all fish-based foods as the main part of the meal.

Examples of meals include poorly glazed tofu, sirtfood omelet, or fried shrimp with buckwheat noodles.

On days 4-7 of the first phase, calorie intake increased to 1,500. This includes two green juices per day and two more foods rich in sirtfood, which you can choose from the book.

Phase 2

Phase 2 lasts two weeks. During this "maintenance" phase, you must continue to lose weight constantly.

There is no Specification for the calorie limit for this phase. Instead, eat three meals full of sirtfood and 1 green juice per day. Again, meals are chosen from the recipes provided in the book.

After the diet

You can repeat these two-steps as much as you want for further weight loss.

However, it is better that you continue to "satiate" your diet after completing these steps by regularly incorporating seed foods into your meals.

There are a lot of Sirtfood Diet books that are full of recipes rich in Sirt foods. You can also include sirt foods in your diet as a snack or in the recipes you already use.

Also, we recommend that you continue to drink green juice every day.

Through this, the Sirtfood diet becomes more of a change in lifestyle than a single diet.

CHAPTER FIVE

7-Day Complete Diet Plan On Sirtfood

Planning a Sirtfood diet menu isn't difficult as long as each Sirtfood Diet and snack have some protein, fiber, complex and a little bit of fat. Eating breakfast will help you start your day with plenty of energy. Don't ruin your breakfast with high-fat and high-calorie foods. Choose some protein and fiber for your breakfast, and it's a good time to eat some fresh fruit.

A mid-morning snack is totally optional. If you eat a larger breakfast, you may not feel hungry until lunchtime. However, if you're feeling a bit hungry and lunch is still two or three hours away, a light mid-morning snack will tide you over without adding a lot of calories.

Lunch is often something you eat at work or school, so it's a great time to pack a sandwich or leftovers that you can heat and eat. Or, if you buy your lunch, choose a healthy clear soup or fresh veggie salad.

A mid-afternoon snack is also optional. Keep it low in calories and eat just enough to keep you from feeling too hungry because dinner is just a couple of hours away.

Dinner is a time when it's easy to over-eat, especially if you haven't eaten much during the day, so watch your portion sizes. Mentally divide your plate into four quarters. One-quarter is for your meat or protein source, one-quarter is for a starch, and the last two-quarters are for green and colorful vegetables or a green salad.

7-Day of Sirtfood Diet Plan

Studying a few examples may make this whole Sirtfood Diet planning thing easier, so here's a full week's worth. You don't need to follow the days in order; you can choose any Sirtfood Diet plan, skip 1 or repeat as you like.

Each day includes three Sirtfood Diets and three snacks and has a healthy balance of fats, and proteins. You'll also get plenty of fiber from whole grains, fruits, vegetables, and legumes.

Every plan includes three Sirtfood Diets and three snacks to keep you feeling satisfied all day long. Some days even include a glass of beer or wine. Feel free to add more water, coffee or herbal tea to any day, but keep in mind that adding cream or sugar also adds calories.

It's OK to swap out similar menu items, but keep cooking methods in mind. Replacing a sirloin steak with grilled chicken is fine, but replacing it with chicken-fried steak isn't going to work because of the breading changes the fat, carb and sodium counts—and the calories.

Finally, you can adjust your calorie intake by eliminating snacks if you want to lose weight or eating larger snacks if you want to gain weight.

Day One

Today's Sirtfood Diet plan contains about 2,250 calories, with 55 percent of those calories coming from carbohydrates, 20 percent fat, and 25 percent from protein. It also has about 34 grams of fiber.

Breakfast

- 1 grapefruit
- Two poached eggs (or fried in a non-stick pan)
- Two slices whole-grain toast with 1 pat butter each
- 1 cup low-fat milk
- 1 cup of black coffee or herbal tea

Snack

- 1 banana
- 1 cup plain yogurt with two tablespoons honey
- Glass of water

Lunch

- Chicken breast (6-ounce portion), baked or roasted (not breaded or fried)
- Large garden salad with tomato and onion with 1 cup croutons, topped with 1 tablespoon oil and vinegar (or salad dressing)
- Glass of water
- (Macronutrients: 425 calories, 44 grams protein, 37 grams carbohydrates, 9 grams fat)

Snack

- 1 cup carrot slices
- Three tablespoon hummus
- One-half piece of pita bread
- Glass of water or herbal tea
- (Macronutrients: 157 calories, 6 grams protein, 25 grams carbohydrates, 5 grams fat)

Dinner

- 1 cup steamed broccoli
- 1 cup of brown rice

- Halibut (four-ounce portion)
- Small garden salad with 1 cup spinach leaves, tomato, and onion topped with two tablespoons oil and vinegar or salad dressing
- 1 glass white wine (regular or dealcoholized)
- Sparkling water with lemon or lime slice

Snack

- 1 cup blueberries
- Two tablespoons whipped cream (the real stuff—whip your own or buy in a can)
- Glass of water
- (Approximately 100 calories, 1 gram protein, 22 grams carbohydrates, 2 grams fat)

Day Two

If you eat this whole menu, you get about 2,150 calories, with 51 percent of those calories coming from carbohydrates, 21 percent from fat, and 28 percent from protein. The Sirtfood Diet plan also has 30 grams of fiber.

Breakfast

- 1 whole-wheat English muffin with two tablespoons peanut butter
- 1 orange
- Large glass (12 ounces) non-fat milk
- 1 cup of black coffee or herbal tea
- (Macronutrients: approximately 521 calories with 27 grams protein, 69 grams carbohydrates, and 18 grams fat)
- **Snack**
- Two oatSirtfood Diet cookies with raisins
- Glass of water, hot tea or black coffee
- (Macronutrients: 130 calories, 2 grams protein, 21 grams carbohydrates, 1 gram fat)

Lunch

- A turkey sandwich (6 ounces of turkey breast meat, large tomato slice, green lettuce and mustard on two slices of whole wheat bread
- 1 cup low-sodium vegetable soup
- Glass of water
- (Macronutrients: 437 calories, 59 grams protein, 37 grams carbohydrates, 6 grams fat)

Snack

- 1 cup (about 30) grapes
- Glass of water or herbal tea
- (Macronutrients: 60 calories, 0.6 grams protein, 12 grams carbohydrates, 0 grams fat)

Dinner

- Five-ounce sirloin steak
- 1 cup mashed potatoes
- 1 cup cooked spinach
- 1 cup green beans
- 1 glass beer (regular, lite or non-alcohol)
- Sparkling water with lemon or lime slice
- (671 calories, 44 grams protein, 63 grams carbohydrates, 18 grams fat)

Snack

- Two slices whole wheat bread with two tablespoons jam (any variety of fruit)
- 1 cup non-fat milk
- Glass of water

- (Approximately 337 calories, 14 grams protein, 66 grams carbohydrates, 3 grams fat)

Day Three

Today's Sirtfood Diet has about 2,260 calories, with 55 percent of those calories coming from carbohydrates, 20 percent from fat, and 25 percent from protein. It also has 50 grams of fiber.

Breakfast

- 1 medium bran muffin
- 1 serving turkey breakfast sausage
- 1 orange
- 1 cup non-fat milk
- 1 cup black coffee or herbal tea
- (Macronutrients: approximately 543 calories with 26 grams protein, 84 grams carbohydrates, and 15 grams fat)

Snack

- 1 fresh pear
- 1 cup of flavored soy milk
- Glass of water, hot tea or black coffee

- (Macronutrients: 171 calories, 6 grams protein, 34 grams carbohydrates, 2 grams fat)

Lunch

- Low sodium chicken noodle soup with six saltine crackers
- 1 medium apple
- Water
- (Macronutrients: 329 calories, 8 grams protein, 38 grams carbohydrates, 17 grams fat)

Snack

- 1 apple
- 1 slice Swiss cheese
- Sparkling water with lemon or lime slice
- (Macronutrients: 151 calories, 5 grams protein, 21 grams carbohydrates, 6 grams fat)

Dinner

8-ounce serving of turkey breast meat

1 cup baked beans

1 cup cooked carrots

1 cup cooked kale

1 glass of wine

(784 calories, 84 grams protein, 76 grams carbohydrates, 3 grams fat)

Snack

1 cup of frozen yogurt

1 cup fresh raspberries

(Approximately 285 calories, 7 grams protein, 52 grams carbohydrates, 7 grams fat)

Day Four

By the end of today, you'll consume about 2,230 calories, with 54 percent of those calories coming from carbohydrates, 24 percent from fat, and 22 percent from protein. You'll also get about 27 grams of fiber.

- **Breakfast**
- 1 cup whole wheat flakes with 1 cup non-fat milk and 1 teaspoon sugar
- 1 banana

- 1 slice whole-grain toast with 1 tablespoon peanut butter
- 1 cup of black coffee or herbal tea
- (Macronutrients: approximately 557 calories with 18 grams protein, 102 grams carbohydrates, and 12 grams fat)

Snack

- 1 cup grapes and 1 tangerine
- Glass of water, hot tea or black coffee
- (Macronutrients: 106 calories, 1 gram protein, 27 grams carbohydrates, 1 gram fat)

Lunch

- Tuna wrap with 1 wheat flour tortilla, one-half can water-packed tuna (drained), 1 tablespoon mayonnaise, lettuce, and sliced tomato
- 1 sliced avocado
- 1 cup non-fat milk
- (Macronutrients: 419 calories, 27 grams protein, 37 grams carbohydrates, 19 grams fat)

Snack

- 1 cup cottage cheese (1-percent fat)
- 1 fresh pineapple slice
- Four graham crackers
- Sparkling water with lemon or lime slice
- (Macronutrients: 323 calories, 29 grams protein, 38 grams carbohydrates, 5 grams fat)

Dinner

- 1 serving lasagna
- Small garden salad with tomatoes and onions topped with 1 tablespoon salad dressing
- 1 cup non-fat milk
- (585 calories, 34 grams protein, 61 grams carbohydrates, 23 grams fat)

Snack

- 1 apple
- 1 cup non-fat milk
- (Approximately 158 calories, 9 grams protein, 31 grams carbohydrates, 1 gram fat)

Day Five

This delicious Sirtfood Diet plan includes three Sirtfood Diets and three snacks and has approximately 2,250 calories, with 53 percent of those calories coming from carbohydrates, 25 percent from fat, and 21 percent from protein. And lots of fiber—over 40 grams.

Breakfast

- 1 piece French toast with 1 tablespoon maple syrup
- 1 scrambled or poached egg
- 1 serving turkey bacon
- 1 cup orange juice
- 1 cup black coffee or herbal tea
- (Macronutrients: approximately 449 calories with 16 grams protein, 57 grams carbohydrates, and 18 grams fat)

Snack

- 1 cup sliced carrots
- 1 cup cauliflower pieces
- Two tablespoons ranch dressing
- Glass of water, hot tea or black coffee

- (Macronutrients: 223 calories, 4 grams protein, 18 grams carbohydrates, 16 grams fat)

Lunch

- Veggie burger on a whole grain bun
- 1 cup northern (or other dry) beans
- 1 cup non-fat milk
- (Macronutrients: 542 calories, 38 grams protein, 85 grams carbohydrates, 8 grams fat)

Snack

- 1 apple
- 1 pita with two tablespoons hummus
- Sparkling water with lemon or lime slice
- (Macronutrients: 202 calories, 5 grams protein, 41 grams carbohydrates, 4 grams fat)

Dinner

- 1 trout filet
- 1 cup green beans
- 1 cup brown rice
- 1 small garden salad with two tablespoons salad dressing

- 1 glass of beer
- Sparkling water with lemon or lime slice
- (634 calories, 27 grams protein, 78 grams carbohydrates, 13 grams fat)

Snack

- 1 cup cottage cheese
- 1 fresh peach
- (Approximately 201 calories, 29 grams protein, 16 grams carbohydrates, 2 grams fat)

Day Six

Today's Sirtfood Diets and snacks have about 2,200 calories, with 55 percent of those calories coming from carbohydrates, 19 percent from fat, and 26 percent from protein. You'll also get about 31 grams fiber.

Breakfast

- 1 cup corn flakes with two teaspoons sugar and 1 cup non-fat milk
- 1 banana
- 1 hard-boiled egg
- 1 cup black coffee or herbal tea

- (Macronutrients: approximately 401 calories with 18 grams protein, 72 grams carbohydrates, and 6 grams fat)

Snack

- 1 cup plain yogurt with 1 tablespoon honey, one-half cup blueberries, and 1 tablespoon almonds
- Glass of water, hot tea or black coffee
- (Macronutrients: 302 calories, 15 grams protein, 46 grams carbohydrates, 8 grams fat)

Lunch

- 1 cup whole wheat pasta with one-half cup red pasta sauce
- Medium garden salad with tomatoes and onions and two tablespoons salad dressing
- Glass of water
- (Macronutrients: 413 calories, 11 grams protein, 67 grams carbohydrates, 12 grams fat)

Snack

- 1 and one-half cup cottage cheese
- 1 fresh peach

- Glass of water
- (Macronutrients: 303 calories, 43 grams protein, 23 grams carbohydrates, 4 grams fat)

Dinner

- Four and one-half ounce serving of pork loin
- Small garden salad with tomatoes and onions topped with two tablespoons oil and vinegar (or salad dressing)
- 1 small baked sweet potato
- 1 cup asparagus
- 1 glass wine (regular or dealcoholized)
- Sparkling water with lemon or lime slice
- (500 calories, 46 grams protein, 35 grams carbohydrates, 10 grams fat)

Snack

- Five graham crackers
- 1 cup non-fat milk
- 1 cup strawberries
- (Approximately 279 calories, 10 grams protein, 50 grams carbohydrates, 3 grams fat)

Day Seven

Today's menu contains about 2,200 calories, with 54 percent of those calories coming from carbohydrates, 22 percent from fat, and 24 percent from protein. There are also 46 grams fiber.

Breakfast

- 1 cup cooked oatSirtfood Diet with one-half cup blueberries, one-half cup non-fat milk, and 1 tablespoon almond slivers
- Two slices turkey bacon
- 1 cup non-fat milk to drink
- 1 cup black coffee or herbal tea
- (Macronutrients: approximately 442 calories with 26 grams protein, 59 grams carbohydrates, and 14 grams fat)

Snack

- 1 cup plain yogurt with 1 tablespoon honey, one-half cup strawberries, and two tablespoons almond slivers
- Glass of water, hot tea or black coffee

- (Macronutrients: 343 calories, 17 grams protein, 41 grams carbohydrates, 13 grams fat)

Lunch

- Six-ounce baked chicken breast
- Large garden salad with tomatoes and onions and two tablespoons salad dressing
- 1 baked sweet potato
- 1 whole-wheat dinner roll.
- Glass of water
- (Macronutrients: 498 calories, 47 grams protein, 63 grams carbohydrates, 6 grams fat)

Snack

- 1 cup raw broccoli florets
- 1 cup raw sliced carrot
- Two tablespoons veggie dip or salad dressing
- 1 fresh peach
- Glass of water
- (Macronutrients: 112 calories, 3 grams protein, 25 grams carbohydrates, 1 gram fat)

Dinner

- 3-ounce serving of baked or grilled salmon
- One-half cup black beans
- 1 cup Swiss chard
- 1 cup brown rice
- 1 whole wheat dinner roll with a pat of butter
- Sparkling water with lemon or lime slice
- (671 calories, 38 grams protein, 91 grams carbohydrates, 19 grams fat)

Snack

- 1 Orange
- (Approximately 62 calories, 1 gram protein, 15 grams carbohydrates, 0 grams fat)
- Planning healthy Sirtfood Diets isn't difficult but if you're not used to it, the planning can take a little practice. The examples we provided should give you a great start.
- Don't feel discouraged if you don't stick to the plan exactly as outlined—it's OK to make variations that fit your lifestyle and needs. Just do your best to incorporate

healthy choices into your day—vegetables, fruit, lean proteins, and legumes, and whole grains are always smart bets.

CHAPTER SIX

Top 20 Sirtfoods

The Sirtfood diet includes a completely new group of Superfoods.

They have been called Sirtfoods because they contain substances that activate Sirtuin or "skinny" genes, the same genes as exercise and fasting.

And there are many Sirt foods that you would expect to see on this list:

1. Bird's eye chilies

2. Buckwheat

3. Capers

4. Celery

5. Cocoa

6. Coffee

7. Extra virgin olive oil

8. Green tea - especially matcha

9. Cabbage

10. Wild celery

11. Give Medjool

12. Parsley

13. Red chicory

14. Red onion

15. Red wine

16. Rocket (rocket)

17. Soy

18. Strawberries

19. Turmeric

20. Walnuts

21. Dark chocolate

Sirt snack food

Here are nine simple Sirtfood snacks that you can reach when you need a SIRT refill.

1 green tea: 1 cup (200 ml / 1 cup) • 1 SIRT 5 per day • 0 calorie

Never underestimate the healthy SIRT enhancement that a cup of green tea can give you. Take as many containers as you can per day; we recommend at least two cups. Not only that, but the SIRTs in green tea is also cumulative, so you can get up to four servings of SIRT per day if you have four cups of green tea or more.

Two red grapes: Ten grapes • 1 SIRT 5 per day • 30 calories.

Another of the straightforward Sirtfood snacks and a low-calorie way to get 1 of your SIRT portions. Keep a basket or two in the fridge and take a handful for breakfast or lunch or both!

Three apples: 1 apple • 1 SIRT 5 per day • 47 calories. Look for an apple as 1 of your easy Sirtfood snacks after lunch. It will also help keep sugar cravings at bay.

Four cocoa: Two teaspoons / 10 g of cocoa • 1 SIRT 5 per day • 33 calories

Try to make a chocolate injection with two teaspoons of cocoa—1 teaspoon of sugar and 30 ml / 2 tbsp of milk. Mix the cocoa and sugar with a little boiling water from the kettle to obtain a smooth paste. Add milk An (almost) instant chocolate with only 68 calories.

Five olives;

Six large black or green olives • 1 SIRT 5 per day • 75 calories

A versatile and easy Sirtfood snack in the afternoon or a snack before dinner. Serve at room temperature for a fuller flavor.

Six blackberries: 15 blackberries • 1 SIRT 5 per day • 32 calories

Another easy-to-store Sirtfood snack in your refrigerator. It is also excellent as a frozen gift.

Seven dark chocolate 85%. Six squares / 20 g / 0.7 oz of chocolate • 1 SIRT 5 per day • 125 calories

Bring your chocolate here! If you prefer 70% dark chocolate, you will need nine squares / 30 g / 1 oz, which will be 180 calories.

Eight pomegranate seeds: 50 g / half sachet • 1 SIRT 5 per day • 50 calories

Easy to take on the go, pomegranate seeds contain a big SIRT bump, and you only need half a 100 g / 3.5 oz packet to get 1 of your SIRT portions.

Blueberries: 25 blueberries (80 g) • 1 of your skirt 5 per day • 36 calories

A large handful of blueberries can also be 1 of your easy Sirtfood snacks.

Ways to try some takeaway foods

Now that you know the facts, here are some easy ways to try eating food.

Green tea

Exchange your maker's tea for green tea. The major difference between the two is that the fresh leaves of the plant are steamed to prepare green tea, while the black leaves are fermented.

Apples

In addition to being classified as a single food, studies have shown that the fruit helps reduce cholesterol and is a good source of fiber, which means it keeps you full For more time,

Parsley

The leaves can be easily cut and sprinkled on dishes from curries to lean steaks. It is also rich in vitamin K, which is good for bones, as well as vitamins A and C.

Blueberries

A wonderful addition to porridge or cereals in the morning, blueberries are rich in vitamin K and also contain vitamin C and fiber.

Strawberries

They are best consumed in summer when they are in season; strawberries are rich in a chemical compound called anthocyanins, which is believed to reduce blood pressure.

Dark chocolate

Studies have shown that cocoa can have links to cardiovascular disease and that dark chocolate is ideal for you than other types because it is generally lower in sugar and fat. But remember that overeating can contribute to weight gain, which is inherently risky.

CHAPTER SEVEN

SIRTFOOD RECIPES

Turmeric Chicken And Kale Salad With Food, Lemon And Honey:

Notes: If prepared in advance, season the salad 10 minutes before serving. Chicken can be replaced with minced meat, minced prawns, or fish. Vegetarians can use chopped mushrooms or cooked quinoa.

Ingredients

For the chicken:

* 1 teaspoon of clarified butter or 1 tablespoon of coconut oil

* ½ medium brown onion, diced

* 250-300 g / 9 ounces minced chicken meat or diced chicken legs

* 1 large garlic clove, diced

* 1 teaspoon of turmeric powder

* 1 teaspoon of lime zest

* ½ lime juice

* ½ teaspoon of salt + pepper

For the salad:

* 6 stalks of broccolini or 2 cups of broccoli flowers

* 2 tablespoons of pumpkin seeds (seeds)

* 3 large cabbage leaves, stems removed and chopped

* ½ sliced avocado

* handful of fresh coriander leaves, chopped

* handful of fresh parsley leaves, chopped

For the dressing:

* 3 tablespoons of lime juice

* 1 small garlic clove, diced or grated

* 3 tablespoons of virgin olive oil (I used 1 tablespoon of avocado oil and * 2 tablespoons of EVO)

* 1 teaspoon of raw honey

* ½ teaspoon whole or Dijon mustard

* ½ teaspoon of sea salt with pepper

Instructions:

1. Heat the coconut oil in a pan. Add the onion and sauté over medium heat for 4-5 minutes, until golden brown. Add the minced chicken and

garlic and stir 2-3 minutes over medium-high heat, separating.

2. Add your turmeric, lime zest, lime juice, salt and pepper, and cook, stirring consistently, for another 3-4 minutes. Set the ground beef aside.

3. While your chicken is cooking, put a small saucepan of water to the boil. Add your broccolini and cook for 2 minutes. Rinse with cold water and cut into 3-4 pieces each.

4. Add the pumpkin seeds to the chicken pan and toast over medium heat for 2 minutes, frequently stirring to avoid burning. Season with a little salt. Set aside. Raw pumpkin seeds are also good to use.

5. Put the chopped cabbage in a salad bowl and pour it over the dressing. Using your hands, mix, and massage the cabbage with the dressing. This

will soften the cabbage, a bit like citrus juice with fish or beef carpaccio: it "cooks" it a little.

6. Finally, mix the cooked chicken, broccolini, fresh herbs, pumpkin seeds, and avocado slices.

Buckwheat spaghetti with chicken cabbage and savory food recipes in mass sauce:

Preparation time: not more than 15 minutes
Cooking time: 15 minutes Total time: 30 minutes

For two people

Ingredients:

For the noodles:

* 2-3 handfuls of cabbage leaves (removed from the stem and cut)

* Buckwheat noodles 150g / 5oz (100% buckwheat, without wheat)

* 3-4 shiitake mushrooms, sliced

* 1 teaspoon of coconut oil or butter

* 1 brown onion, finely chopped

* 1 medium chicken breast, sliced or diced

* 1 long red pepper, thinly sliced (seeds in or out depending on how hot you like it)

* 2 large garlic cloves, diced

* 2-3 tablespoons of Tamari sauce (gluten-free soy sauce)

For the miso dressing:

* 1 tablespoon and a half of fresh organic miso

* 1 tablespoon of Tamari sauce

* 1 tablespoon of extra virgin olive oil

* 1 tablespoon of lemon or lime juice

* 1 teaspoon of sesame oil (optional)

Instructions

1. Boil a medium saucepan of water. Add the black cabbage and cook 1 minute, until it is wilted. Remove and reserve, but reserve the water and return to boiling. Add your soba noodles and cook according to the directions on the package (usually about 5 minutes). Rinse with cold water and reserve.

2. In the meantime, fry the shiitake mushrooms in a little butter or coconut oil (about a teaspoon) for 2-3 minutes, until its color is lightly browned on each side. Sprinkle with sea salt and reserve.

3. In that same pan, heat more coconut oil or lard over medium-high heat. Fry the onion and chili for 2-3 minutes, then add the chicken pieces. Cook 5 minutes on medium heat, stirring a few times, then add the garlic, tamari sauce, and a little water. Cook for another 2-3 minutes,

stirring continuously until your chicken is cooked.

4. Finally, add the cabbage and soba noodles and stir the chicken to warm it.

5. Stir the miso sauce and sprinkle the noodles at the end of the cooking, in this way you will keep alive all the beneficial probiotics in the miso.

Asia King Jumped Jamp With Lunch
Lunch:

- 150 g / 5 oz of raw shelled prawns, not chopped

- Two teaspoons of tamari (you can use soy sauce if you don't avoid gluten)

- Two teaspoons of extra virgin olive oil

- 75 g / 2.6 oz soba (buckwheat pasta)

- 1 garlic clove, finely chopped

- 1 bird's eye chili, finely chopped

- 1 teaspoon finely chopped fresh ginger.

- 20 g / 0.7 oz of sliced red onions

- 40 g / 1.4 oz of celery, cut and sliced

- 75 g / 2.6 oz of chopped green beans

- 50 g / 1.7 oz of chopped cabbage

- 100 ml / ½ cup of chicken broth

- 5 g celery or celery leaves

Instructions:

Heat a pan over high heat, then cook the prawns in 1 teaspoon of tamari and 1 teaspoon of oil for 2-3 minutes. Transfer the prawns to a plate. Clean the pan with kitchen paper as it will be reused.

Cook your noodles in boiling water for 5-8 minutes or as indicated on the package. Drain and set aside.

Meanwhile, fry the garlic, chili and ginger, red onion, celery, beans, and cabbage in the remaining oil over medium-high heat for 2-3 minutes. Add your broth and allow it to boil, then simmer for a minute or two, until the vegetables are cooked but crunchy.

Add shrimp, noodles and celery/celery leaves to the pan, bring to a boil again, then remove from the heat and serve.

Buckwheat Pasta Salad:

- Serves 1
- 50 g / 1.7 oz buckwheat pasta
- large handful of rocket
- a small handful of basil leaves
- Eight cherry tomatoes halved
- 1/2 avocado, diced
- Ten olives
- 1 tbsp extra olive virgin oil
- 20 g / 0.70 oz pine nuts

combine all the ingredients except your pine nuts. Arrange your combination on a plate, then scatter the pine nuts over the top.

Greek Salad Skewers:

- Two wooden skewers, soaked in water for 30 minutes before use

- Eight large black olives

- Eight cherry tomatoes

- 1 yellow pepper, cut into eight squares.

- ½ red onion, you can cut in half and separated into eight pieces

- 100 g / 3.5 oz (about 10cm) cucumber, cut into four slices and halved

- 100 g / 3.5 oz feta, cut into eight cubes

For the dressing:

- 1 tbsp extra olive virgin oil

- Juice of ½ lemon

- 1 tsp of your balsamic vinegar

- ½ clove garlic, ensure it peeled and crushed

- basil leaves chopped (or ½ tsp dried mixed herbs to replace basil and oregano)

- oregano leaves,
- salt and grounded black pepper

- 1 blend each skewer with the salad ingredients in the order

- 2 Put all your dressing ingredients into a bowl and mix thoroughly. Pour over the skewers.

Kale, Edamame And Tofu Curry:

- 1 tbsp rapeseed oil
- 1 large onion, chopped
- Four cloves garlic, peeled and grated
- 1 large thumb (7cm) fresh ginger, peeled and grated
- 1 red chili, deseeded and thinly sliced
- 1/2 tsp ground turmeric
- 1/4 tsp cayenne pepper
- 1 tsp paprika
- 1/2 tsp ground cumin
- 1 tsp salt
- 250 g / 9 oz dried red lentils
- 1 liter boiling water
- 50 g / 1.7 oz frozen soya beans
- 200 g / 7 oz firm tofu, chopped into cubes
- Two tomatoes, roughly chopped
- Juice of 1 lime
- 200 g / 7 oz kale leaves stalk removed and torn

1 Put the oil in a pan over low heat. Add your onion and cook for 5 minutes before adding the

garlic, ginger, and chili and cooking for a further 2 minutes. Add your turmeric, cayenne, paprika, cumin, and salt and Stir through before adding the red lentils and stirring again.

2 Pour in the boiling water and allow it to simmer for 10 minutes, reduce the heat and cook for about 20-30 minutes until the curry has a thick '•porridge' consistency.

3 Add your tomatoes, tofu and soya beans and cook for a further 5 minutes. Add your kale leaves and lime juice and cook until the kale is just tender.

Chocolate Cupcakes With Matcha Icing:

- 150g / 5 oz self-raising flour

- 200 g / 7 oz caster sugar

- 60 g / 2.1 oz cocoa

- ½ tsp salt

- ½ tsp fine espresso coffee, decaf if preferred

- 120 ml / ½ cup milk

- ½ tsp vanilla extract

- 50 ml / ¼ cup vegetable oil

- 1 egg

- 120 ml / ½ cup of water

- **For the icing:**

- 50 g / 1.7 oz butter,

- 50 g / 1.7 oz icing sugar

- 1 tbsp matcha green tea powder

- ½ tsp vanilla bean paste

- 50 g / 1.7 oz soft cream cheese

• heat the oven and Line a cupcake tin with paper

• Put the flour, sugar, cocoa, salt, and coffee powder in a large bowl and mix well.

• Add milk, vanilla extract, vegetable oil, and egg to dry ingredients and use an electric mixer to beat until well combined. Gently pour the boiling water slowly and beat on low speed until completely combined. Use the high speed to beat for another minute to add air to the dough. The dough is much more liquid than a normal cake mix. Have faith; It will taste fantastic!

• Arrange the dough evenly between the cake boxes. Each cake box must not be more than ¾ full. Bake for 15-18 minutes, until the dough resumes when hit. Remove from oven and allow to cool completely before icing.

• To make the icing, beat your butter and icing sugar until they turn pale and smooth. Add the matcha powder and vanilla and mix again. Add the cream cheese and beat until it is smooth. Pipe or spread on the cakes.

Sesame Chicken Salad:

- 1 tablespoon of sesame seeds

- 1 cucumber, peeled, halved lengthwise, without a teaspoon, and sliced.

- 100 g / 3.5 oz cabbage, chopped

- 60 g pak choi, finely chopped

- ½ red onion, thinly sliced

- Large parsley (20 g / 0.7 oz), chopped.

- 150 g / 5 oz cooked chicken, minced

- For the dressing:

- 1 tablespoon of extra virgin olive oil

- 1 teaspoon of sesame oil

- 1 lime juice

1 teaspoon of light honey

2 teaspoons soy sauce

1 Toast your sesame seeds in a dry pan for 2 minutes until they become slightly golden and fragrant. Transfer to a plate to cool.

2 In a small bowl, mix olive oil, sesame oil, lime juice, honey, and soy sauce to prepare the dressing.

3 Place the cucumber, black cabbage, pak choi, red onion, and parsley in a large bowl and mix gently. Pour over the dressing and mix again.

4 Distribute the salad between two dishes and complete with the shredded chicken. Sprinkle with sesame seeds just before serving.

Mushroom Scramble Eggs:

- Two eggs

- 1 tsp ground turmeric

- 1 tsp mild curry powder

- 20 g / 0.70 oz kale, roughly chopped

- 1 tsp extra virgin olive oil

- ½ bird's eye chili, thinly sliced

- a handful of mushrooms, thinly sliced

- 5 g / 1 tsp of parsley finely chopped

- * optional * Add a seed mix for garnish and a little rooster sauce for flavor

Instructions:

Mix the turmeric and curry powder and add a little water until you get a light paste.

Steam the cabbage for 2-3 minutes.

Heat the oil in a pan over medium heat and fry the red pepper and mushrooms for 2-3 minutes until they begin to brown and soften.

Aromatic chicken breasts with cabbage, red onion and sauce:

- 120 g / 4 oz boneless skinless chicken breast

- 2 teaspoons of turmeric powder

- ¼ lemon juice

- 1 tablespoon of extra virgin olive oil

- 50 g / 1.7 oz of chopped cabbage

- 20 g / 0.7 oz of red onion, sliced

- 1 teaspoon chopped fresh ginger

- 50 g / 1.7 oz of buckwheat

Instructions:

To prepare the sauce, remove the eye from the tomato and cut it very finely, taking care to keep as much liquid as possible. Mix with the chili pepper, capers, parsley, and lemon juice. You could put everything in a blender, but the result is slightly different.

Heat the oven to 220 ° C / 430 ° F / gas 7. Marinate the chicken breast in 1 teaspoon of turmeric, lemon juice and a little oil. Leave to act for 5-10 minutes.

Cook the buckwheat according to the directions on the package with the remaining teaspoon of turmeric. Serve with chicken, vegetables and sauce.

Smoked Salmon Omelet:

Try this quick and easy Sirtfood dish full of flavor and goodness.

serves:

one

- Preparation time:
- 5-10 minutes
- ingredients
- 2 medium eggs
- 100 g / 3.5 oz of smoked salmon, sliced
- 1/2 teaspoon capers
- 10 g / 0.35 oz of chopped rocket
- 1 teaspoon minced parsley
- 1 teaspoon of extra virgin olive oil

Method

Break the eggs in a bowl and beat well. Add salmon, capers, arugula and parsley.

Heat the olive oil in a non-stick pan until it is hot but not smoking. Add the egg mixture and, using a spatula or a slice of fish, move the mixture around the pan until it is uniform. Reduce the heat and let the omelette cook. Slide the spatula around the edges and roll or fold the tortilla in half to serve.

Heat an ovenproof skillet until hot, then add the marinated chicken and cook for about a minute on each side, until lightly browned, then transfer to the oven (place in a skillet if the skillet is not ovenproof) for 8-10 minutes or until cooked. Remove from the oven, cover with aluminum foil and let rest for 5 minutes before serving.

Meanwhile, cook the black cabbage in a steamer for 5 minutes. Fry the red onions and ginger in a little oil until soft but not colored, then add the cooked cabbage and fry for another minute.

Green Tea Smoothie:

This super-healthy smoothie uses matcha powder, which is a highly concentrated Japanese green tea. It can be found in specialist Asian or tea shops.

Serves 2 • Ready in 3 minutes

- Two ripe bananas
- 250 ml / 1 cup of milk
- 2 tsp matcha green tea powder
- 1/2 tsp vanilla bean paste (not extract) or a small scrape of the seeds from a vanilla pod
- Six ice cubes
- 2 tsp honey

Simply blend all the ingredients in a blender and serve in two glasses.

Sirt Food Miso Marinated Cod, Stir-Fried Greens & Sesame:

- 20 g / 0.70 oz miso

- 1 tbsp mirin

- 1 tbsp extra virgin olive oil

- 200 g / 7 oz skinless cod fillet

- 20 g / 0.70 oz red onion, sliced

- 40 g / 1.4 oz celery, sliced

- 1 garlic clove, finely chopped

- 1 bird's eye chili, finely chopped

- 1 tsp finely chopped fresh ginger

- 60 g / 2.1 oz green beans

- 50 g / 1.7 oz kale, roughly chopped

- 1 tsp sesame seeds

- 5g / 1 tsp parsley, roughly chopped

- 1 tbsp tamari

- 30 g / 1 oz buckwheat

- 1 tsp ground turmeric

Instructions:

Mix the miso, mirin, and 1 teaspoon of the oil. Rub all over the cod and leave to marinate for 30 minutes. Heat the oven to 220°C/gas 7.

Bake the cod for 10 minutes.

Meanwhile, heat a large frying pan or wok with the remaining oil. Add the onion and stir-fry for a few minutes, then add the celery, garlic, chili, ginger, green beans, and kale. Toss and fry until the kale is tender and cooked through. You may need to add a little water to the pan to aid the cooking process.

Cook the buckwheat according to the packet instructions with the turmeric for 3 minutes.

Add the sesame seeds, parsley, and tamari to the stir-fry and serve with the greens and fish.

Raspberry and Blackcurrant Jelly:

Making a jelly in advance is a great way to prepare the fruit so that it is ready to eat first thing in the morning.

Serves 2 • Ready in 15 minutes + setting time

- 100 g / 3.5 oz raspberries washed
- 2 leaves gelatine
- 100 g / 3.5 oz blackcurrants washed and stalks removed
- 2 tbsp granulated sugar
- 300 ml / 1 and ¼ cup water

1 Arrange the raspberries in two serving dishes/glasses/molds. Put the gelatine leaves in a bowl of cold water to soften.

2 Place the blackcurrants in a small pan with the sugar and 100ml / ½ cup water and bring to the boil. Simmer vigorously for 5 minutes and then remove from the heat. Leave to stand for 2 minutes.

3 Squeeze out excess water from the gelatine leaves and add them to the saucepan. Stir until fully dissolved, then stir in the rest of the water. Pour the liquid into the prepared dishes and refrigerate to set. The jellies should be ready in about 3-4 hours or overnight.

Apple Pancakes with Blackcurrant Compote:

These pancakes are decadent but healthy—a great lazy morning treat.

Serves 4 • Ready in 20 minutes

- 75g / 2.6 oz porridge oats sirtfood recipes
- 125g / 4.4 oz plain flour
- 1 tsp baking powder
- 2 tbsp caster sugar
- Pinch of salt
- Two apples, peeled, cored and cut into small pieces
- 300 ml / 1 and ¼ cup semi-skimmed milk
- Two egg whites
- 2 tsp light olive oil

For the compote:

- 120 g / 4.2 oz blackcurrants washed and stalks removed
- 2 tbsp caster sugar
- 3 tbsp water

1 First, make the compote. Place the blackcurrants, sugar, and water in a small pan. Bring up to a simmer and cook for 10-15 minutes.

2 Place the oats, flour, baking powder, caster sugar and salt in a large bowl and mix well. Stir in the apple and then whisk in the milk a little at a time until you have a smooth mixture. Whisk the egg whites to stiff peaks and then fold into the pancake batter. Transfer the batter to a jug.

3 Heat 1/2 tsp oil in a non-stick frying pan on medium-high heat and pour in approximately

one-quarter of the batter. Cook on both sides until golden brown. Remove and repeat to make four pancakes.

4 Serve the pancakes with the blackcurrant compote drizzled over.

SIRT Fruit Salad:

This fruit salad is packed full of the best fruit SIRTs.

Serves 1 • Ready in 10 minutes

- ½ cup freshly made green tea
- 1 tsp honey
- 1 orange halved
- 1 apple, cored and roughly chopped
- Ten red seedless grapes
- Ten blueberries

1 Stir the honey into half a cup of green tea. When dissolved, add the juice of half the orange. Leave to cool.

2 Chop the other half of the orange and place in a bowl together with the chopped apple, grapes,

and blueberries. Pour over the cooled tea and leave to steep for a few minutes before serving.

Sirtfood Bites:

1. 120 g / 4.2 oz walnuts
2. 30 g / 1 oz dark chocolate (85 percent cocoa solids), broken into pieces; or cocoa nibs
3. 250 g / 9 oz Medjool dates pitted
4. 1 tbsp cocoa powder
5. 1 tbsp ground turmeric
6. 1 tbsp extra virgin olive oil
7. the scraped seeds of 1 vanilla pod or 1 tsp vanilla extract
8. 1–2 tbsp water

INSTRUCTIONS

Place the walnuts and chocolate in a food processor and process until you have a fine powder.

Add all the other ingredients except the water and blend until the mixture forms a ball. You may or may not have to add the water depending on the consistency of the mixture – you don't want it to be too sticky.

Using your hands, form the mixture into bite-sized balls and refrigerate in an airtight container for at least 1 hour before eating them.

You could roll some of the balls in some more cocoa or desiccated coconut to achieve a different finish if you like.

They will keep for up to 1 week in your fridge.

Sirt Muesli:

Ingredients:

- 20 g / 0.70 oz buckwheat flakes

- 10 g / 0.35 oz buckwheat puffs

- 15 g / 0.5 oz coconut flakes or desiccated coconut

- 40 g / 1.4 oz Medjool dates, pitted and chopped

- 15 g / 0.5 oz walnuts, chopped

- 10 g / 0.35 oz cocoa nibs

- 100 g / 3.5 oz strawberries, hulled and chopped

- 100 g / 3.5 oz plain Greek yogurt (or vegan alternative, such as soya or coconut yogurt)

Instructions:

Mix all of the above ingredients, only adding the yogurt and strawberries before serving if you are making it in bulk.

Chinese-Style Pork With Pak Choi:
Ingredients

- 400g / 14 oz firm tofu, cut into large cubes
- 1 tbsp cornflour
- 1 tbsp water
- 125ml / ½ cup chicken stock
- 1 tbsp rice wine
- 1 tbsp tomato purée
- 1 tsp brown sugar
- 1 tbsp soy sauce
- 1 clove garlic, peeled and crushed
- 1 thumb (5cm) fresh ginger, peeled and grated 1 tbsp rapeseed oil
- 100 g / 3.5 oz shiitake mushrooms, sliced
- 1 shallot, peeled and sliced
- 200 g / 7 oz pak choi or Choi sum, cut into thin slices 400g / 14 oz pork mince (10% fat)

- 100 g / 3.5 oz beansprouts
- Large handful (20g) parsley, chopped

Here's how:

Place the tofu on kitchen paper, cover with other kitchen paper and set aside.

In a small bowl, mix the cornmeal and water together, removing all lumps. Add chicken broth, rice wine, tomato puree, brown sugar and soy sauce. Add the minced garlic and ginger and mix together.

In a pan or wok, heat the oil over high heat. Add the shiitake mushrooms and fry them for 2-3 minutes until cooked and shiny. Remove the mushrooms from the pan with a perforated spoon and set aside. Add the tofu to the pan and brown until golden brown on all sides. Remove with a perforated spoon and set aside.

Add the shallot and pak choi to the wok, brown for 2 minutes, then add the minced meat. Cook until the minced meat is completely cooked, then add the sauce, reduce the heat by 1 notch and let the sauce penetrate around the meat for a minute or two. Add beans, shiitake mushrooms and tofu to the pan and heat. Remove from the heat, mix the parsley and serve immediately.

Tuscan Bean Stew:

ingredients

- 1 tablespoon of extra virgin olive oil
- 50 g / 1.7 oz of red onion, finely chopped
- 30 g / 1 oz of carrots, peeled and finely chopped sirtfood recipes
- 30 g / 1 oz of celery, finely chopped and chopped
- A clove of garlic, finely chopped
- ½ hot pepper, finely chopped (optional)
- 1 teaspoon of Provence herbs
- 200 ml / 1 cup of vegetable broth
- 1 x 400 g / 14 oz of canned chopped Italian tomatoes
- 1 teaspoon tomato sauce
- 200 g / 7 oz of canned mixed beans
- 50 g / 1.7 oz of chopped cabbage
- 1 spoonful of chopped parsley

- 40 g / 1.4 oz of buckwheat

Cook the buckwheat according to the directions on the package with the remaining teaspoon of turmeric. Serve with chicken, vegetables, and sauce.

Smoked Salmon Omelette:

Try this quick and easy Sirtfood dish full of flavor and goodness.

ingredients

- 2 medium eggs
- 100 g / 3.5 oz smoked salmon, sliced
- 1/2 teaspoon of capers
- 10 g / 0.35 oz chopped rocket
- 1 teaspoon of chopped parsley
- 1 teaspoon of extra virgin olive oil

Method

Break the eggs into a bowl and beat well. Add salmon, capers, arugula, and parsley.

Heat the olive oil in a nonstick skillet until hot but not smoking. Add the egg mixture and, using a spatula or a slice of fish, move the mixture around the pan until smooth. Reduce the heat and let the omelette cook. Slide spatula around edges and roll or fold tortilla in half to serve.

Arrange the salad leaves on a large plate. Mix all the remaining ingredients and serve on top of the leaves.

Chip Granola:

Chocolate at breakfast! Be sure to serve with a cup of green tea to give you plenty of SIRTs. The rice malt syrup can be substituted with maple syrup if you prefer.

Serves 8 • Ready in 30 minutes

- 200 g / 7 oz jumbo oats
- 50 g / 1.7 oz pecans, roughly
- chopped
- 3 tbsp light olive oil
- 20 g / 0.70 oz butter
- 1 tbsp dark brown sugar
- 2 tbsp rice malt syrup
- 60 g / 2.1 oz good-quality (70%)
- dark chocolate chips

1 Preheat the oven to 160°C / 320°F (140°C/ 280°F fan / Gas 3). Line a large baking tray with a silicone sheet or baking parchment.

2 Mix the oats and pecans in a large bowl. In a small non-stick pan, gently heat the olive oil, butter, brown sugar, and rice malt syrup until the butter has melted and the sugar and syrup have dissolved. Do not allow to boil. Pour the syrup over the oats and stir thoroughly until the oats are fully covered.

3 Distribute the granola over the baking tray, spreading right into the corners. Leave clumps of the mixture with spacing rather than an even spread. Bake in the oven for 20 minutes until just tinged golden brown at the edges. Remove from the oven and leave to cool on the tray completely.

4 When cool, break up any bigger lumps on the tray with your fingers and then mix in the

chocolate chips. Scoop or pour the granola into an airtight tub or jar. The granola will keep for at least two weeks.

Fragrant Asian Hotpot:

- 1 tsp tomato purée
- 1-star anise, crushed (or 1/4 tsp ground anise)
- Small handful (10 g / 0.35 oz) parsley, stalks finely chopped
- Small handful (1Og) coriander, stalks finely chopped
- Juice of 1/2 lime
- 500 ml / 2 cups chicken stock, fresh or made with 1 cube
- 1/2 carrot, peeled and cut into matchsticks
- 50 g / 1.7 oz broccoli, cut into small florets
- 50 g / 1.7 oz beansprouts
- 1OOg raw tiger prawns
- 1OOg firm tofu, chopped
- 50 g / 1.7 oz rice noodles, cooked according to packet instructions

- 50 g / 1.7 oz cooked water chestnuts, drained
- 20 g / 0.70 oz sushi ginger, chopped
- 1 tbsp good-quality miso paste

Place the tomato purée, star anise, parsley stalks, coriander stalks, lime juice, and chicken stock in a large pan and bring to a simmer for 10 minutes.

Add the carrot, broccoli, prawns, tofu, noodles, and water chestnuts and simmer gently until the prawns are cooked through. Remove from the heat and stir in the sushi ginger and miso paste.

Serve sprinkled with the parsley and coriander leaves.

Lamb, Butternut Squash And Date Tagine:

Ingredients

- Two tablespoons olive oil
- 1 red onion, sliced
- 2cm ginger, grated
- Three garlic cloves, grated or crushed
- 1 teaspoon chili flakes (or to taste)
- Two teaspoons cumin seeds
- 1 cinnamon stick
- Two teaspoons ground turmeric
- 800 g / 28 oz lamb neck fillet, cut into 2cm chunks
- ½ teaspoon salt
- 100 g / 3.5 oz Medjool dates, pitted and chopped

- 400g / 14 oz tin chopped tomatoes, plus half a can of water
- 500 g / 18 oz butternut squash, chopped into 1cm cubes
- 400g / 14 oz tin chickpeas, drained
- Two tablespoons fresh coriander (plus extra for garnish)
- Buckwheat, couscous, flatbreads or rice to serve

Method

1. Preheat your oven to 140C.

2. Drizzle about two tablespoons olive oil in a large saucepan or cast iron saucepan. Add the sliced onion and simmer, with the lid on, for about 5 minutes, until the onions soften but are not browned.

3. Add the grated garlic and ginger, chili, cumin, cinnamon, and turmeric. Mix well and cook for

another minute without the lid. Add a little water if it dries too much.

4. Then add the pieces of lamb. Mix well to coat the meat with onion and spices and then add the salt, the chopped dates and the tomatoes, plus approximately half a can of water (100-200 ml / 1 cup).

5. Bring the tajine to a boil, then put the lid on and put it in the preheated oven for 1 hour and 15 minutes.

6. Thirty minutes before the end of the cooking time, add the chopped butternut squash and drained chickpeas. Mix everything, replace the lid and return to the oven during the last 30 minutes of cooking.

7. When the tagine is done, remove it from the oven and mix it with the chopped coriander. Serve with buckwheat, couscous, focaccia, or basmati rice.

If you don't have a ovenproof saucepan or cast iron saucepan, just cook the labels in a regular saucepan until you have to go to the oven, and then transfer the labels to a saucepan with a normal lid before putting them in the oven. Add another 5 minutes of cooking to allow the saucepan to heat up.

Prawn Arrabbiata:

ingredients

- 125-150 g / 4.5-5.5 oz of raw or cooked prawns (ideally prawns)
- 65 g / 2.3oz buckwheat pasta
- 1 tablespoon of extra virgin olive oil
- For arrabbiata sauce
- 40 g / 1.4 oz red onion, finely chopped
- 1 garlic clove, finely minced
- 30 g / 1 oz celery, finely chopped
- 1 chile on view, finely chopped
- 1 teaspoon mixed dried herbs
- 1 teaspoon of extra virgin olive oil
- 2 tablespoons of white wine (optional)
- 400 g / 14 oz canned chopped tomatoes

- 1 tablespoon of chopped parsley

Method

1. Fry the onion, garlic, celery, and red pepper and dried herbs in the oil over medium-low heat for 1-2 minutes. Turn the heat on average, add the wine and cook for 1 minute. Add the tomatoes and bring the sauce to a boil over medium-low heat for 20-30 minutes, until it has a pleasant and rich consistency. If you feel the sauce is getting too thick, just add a little water.

2. While the sauce is cooking, bring a pan to the boil with water and cook the pasta according to the directions on the package. If cooked to your liking, drain, mix with olive oil and store in a pan until necessary.

3. If you are using raw prawns, add them to the sauce and cook for another 3-4 minutes, until they become pink and opaque, add the parsley and serve. If you use cooked prawns, add them with parsley, boil the sauce and serve.

4. Add the cooked pasta to the sauce, mix well but carefully and serve.

Turmeric Baked Salmon:

Ingredients

- 125-150 g / 4.5- 5.5 oz Skinned Salmon
- 1 tsp Extra virgin olive oil
- 1 tsp ground turmeric
- ¼ Juice of a lemon
- For the spicy celery
- 1 tsp Extra virgin olive oil
- 40 g / 1.4 oz Red onion, finely chopped
- 60 g / 2 oz Tinned green lentils
- 1 Garlic clove, finely chopped
- 1 cm fresh ginger, finely chopped
- 1 Bird's eye chili, finely chopped
- 150 g / 1.7 oz Celery, cut into 2cm lengths
- 1 tsp Mild curry powder
- 130 g / 4.5 oz Tomato, cut into eight wedges

- 100 ml / ½ cup Chicken or vegetable stock

- 1 tbsp Chopped parsley

Method

Heat oven to 200 ° C / 390 ° F / gas 6.

Start with hot celery. Heat a frying pan over medium-low heat, add the olive oil, then the onion, garlic, ginger, chilli and celery. Fry gently for 2-3 minutes or until softened but not colored, then add the curry powder and cook for another minute.

Add the tomatoes, then the broth and lentils and simmer for 10 minutes. You may want to increase or decrease the cooking time, depending on how much you like the crispy celery.

Meanwhile, mix the turmeric, oil, and lemon juice and rub the salmon. # Place on a baking sheet and cook for 8-10 minutes.

To finish, mix the parsley through the celery and serve with the salmon.

Coronation Chicken Salad:

Ingredients

- 75 g / 2.6 oz Natural yogurt
- 1/4 lemon juice
- 1 teaspoon minced coriander
- 1 teaspoon of turmeric powder
- 1/2 teaspoon mild curry
- 100 g / 3.5 oz cooked chicken breast, cut into small pieces
- 6 half walnuts, finely chopped
- 1 Medjool date, finely chopped
- 20 g / 0.7 oz red onion, diced
- 1 chili bird's eye
- 40 g / 1.4 oz of rocket, a
- serve

Method

Mix the yogurt, lemon juice, coriander, and spices in a bowl. Add all the remaining ingredients and serve on a bed of the rocket.

Baked Potatoes With Spicy Chicken Stir:

A species of Mexican mole meets North African tagine, this spicy chickpea stew is incredibly delicious and an excellent ingredient for baked potatoes, as well as being vegetarian, vegan, gluten-free and milk-free. And it contains chocolate.

Ingredients

- 4-6 baking potatoes, pricked all over
- Two tablespoons olive oil
- Two red onions, finely chopped
- Four cloves garlic, grated or crushed
- 2cm ginger, grated
- ½ -2 teaspoons chili flakes
- Two tablespoons cumin seeds
- Two tablespoons turmeric

- Splash of water

- 2 x 400g / 14 oz tins chopped tomatoes

- Two tablespoons unsweetened cocoa powder (or cacao)

- 2 x 400g / 14 oz tins chickpeas (or kidney beans if you prefer) including the chickpea water DON'T DRAIN!!

- Two yellow peppers (or whatever color you prefer!), chopped into bitesize pieces

- Two tablespoons parsley plus extra for garnish

- Salt and pepper to taste (optional)

- Side salad (optional)

Method

1. Preheat the oven to 200 ° C / 390 ° F, meanwhile you can prepare all its ingredients.

2. When the oven is hot enough, put the potatoes in the oven and cook for 1 hour or until done as desired.

3. Once the potatoes are in the oven, add the olive oil and the chopped red onion in a large saucepan and cook gently, with the lid on for 5 minutes, until the onions are soft but not browned.

4. Remove the lid and add garlic, ginger, cumin, and chili. Simmer for another minute, then add the turmeric and a little water and cook for another minute, being careful not to let the pan dry out too much.

5. Then add the tomatoes, cocoa powder (or cocoa), chickpeas (including chickpea water), and yellow pepper. Bring to a boil, then simmer for 45 minutes until the sauce is thick and oily (but don't let it burn!). The stew should be done at about the same time as the potatoes.

6. Finally, add the two tablespoons of parsley and, if desired, salt and pepper and serve the stew on top of the baked potatoes, perhaps with a simple salad.

Grape And Melon Juice:

- 125 calories
- 2 of your SIRT 5 per day
- Doses for 1 • Ready in 2 minutes
- ½ cucumber, peeled if you prefer, halved, sown and chopped
- 30 g / 1 oz of young spinach leaves removed
- 100 g / 3.5 oz of seedless red grapes
- 100 g / 3.5 oz melon, peeled, sown and cut into pieces
- 1 Stir in a blender or blender until smooth.

Kale And Red Onion Dhal With Buckwheat:

This Kale and Red Onion Dhal with Buckwheat are quick and very easy to make and naturally gluten-free, dairy-free, vegetarian, and vegan.

Ingredients:

- 1 tablespoon olive oil

- 1 small red onion, sliced.

- Three garlic cloves, grated or crushed

- 2 cm ginger, grated

- 1 bird's eye chili, deseeded and finely chopped (more if you like things hot!)

- Two teaspoons turmeric

- Two teaspoons of Garam Masala

- 160 g / 5.5 oz of red lentils

- 400 ml / 2 cup of coconut milk

- 200 ml / 1 cup of water

- 100 g / 3.5 oz of cabbage (or spinach would be an excellent alternative)

- 160 g / 5.5 oz of buckwheat (or brown rice)

METHOD

1. Put the olive oil in a deep saucepan and add the sliced onion and cook.

2. Add the ginger, pepper, garlic, and cook for another minute.

3. Add fresh turmeric, garam masala, and a little water and cook for another minute.

4. Add the red lentils, coconut milk, and 200 ml / 1 cup of water.

5. Mix everything well and cook for 20 minutes on low heat with the lid on. Stir continuously and add a little more water if the Dhal starts attacking.

6. After 20 minutes, add the cabbage, mix well, and put the lid back on, cook for another 5 minutes (1-2 minutes if you use spinach instead!)

7. 15 minutes before the curry is ready, put the buckwheat in a medium saucepan, and add a lot of boiling water. Allow the water to a boil again and cook for 10 minutes (or a little more if you prefer your buckwheat to be softer. Drain the buckwheat in a sieve and serve with the dhal).

Carbilled Meat, Garlic Lime And Herbal Potato:

- 100 g / 3.5 oz potatoes, peeled and cut into 2 cm cubes

- 1 tablespoon of extra virgin olive oil

- 5 g / 1 tsp of parsley finely chopped

- 50 g / 1.7 oz red onion, cut into slices

- 50 g / 1.7 oz sliced cabbage

- A clove of garlic finely minced

- Beef tenderloin 120-150 g / 4-5 oz x 3.5 cm thick or sirloin steak 2 cm thick

- 40 ml / 3 tbsp of red wine

- 150 ml / ½ cup beef broth

- 1 teaspoon of tomato sauce

- 1 teaspoon of cornmeal, dissolved in 1 tablespoon of water

Instructions:

Heat oven to 220 ° C / 430 ° F / gas 7.

Put your potatoes in a saucepan with boiling water, boil and cook for 4-5 minutes, then drain. Place in a pan with a teaspoon of oil and roast in the hot oven for 35-45 minutes. Rotate the potatoes every 10 minutes to ensure it is cooked well. After cooking, remove from the oven, sprinkle with the chopped parsley, and mix well.

Fry the onion in 1 teaspoon of oil over medium heat for 5-7 minutes, until smooth and well caramelized. Keeping warm Steam the cabbage for 2-3 minutes, then drain. Gently fry the garlic in ½ teaspoon of oil for 1 minute until it softens but is not colored. Add cabbage and fry for another 1-2 minutes, until tender. Keeping warm

Heat an ovenproof skillet over high heat until smoke comes out. Spread the meat in half a teaspoon of oil and fry in the hot skillet over medium-high heat depending on how you like the meat. If you prefer your meat medium, it would be better to brown the meat and then transfer the pan to an oven at 220 ° C / 430 ° F / seven gas and finish cooking this way for the prescribed times.

Remove meat from skillet and keep to rest. Add the wine in the hot pan to remove the meat remnants: bubbles to cut the wine in half until you get syrup and a concentrated flavor.

Add the broth and tomato puree to the meat pan and bring to a boil, then add the cornmeal paste to thicken the sauce, adding it little by little until you get the desired consistency. Mix any of the juices from the rested steak and serve with roasted potatoes, black cabbage, onion rings, and red wine sauce.

If you enjoyed this book, please let me know your thoughts by leaving a short review on Amazon. Thank you